# THE TYPE 2 DIABETES DESSERTS COOKBOOK

Also by Lois M. Soneral

*The Type II Diabetes Cookbook*

# THE TYPE 2 DIABETES DESSERTS COOKBOOK

## Lois M. Soneral

### foreword by Charles L. Chavez, M.D.

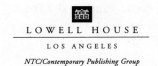

LOWELL HOUSE

LOS ANGELES

*NTC/Contemporary Publishing Group*

Library of Congress Cataloging-in-Publication Data

Soneral, Lois M.
    The type 2 diabetes desserts cookbook / Lois M. Soneral ;
foreword by Charles L. Chavez.
        p.    cm.
    ISBN 0-7373-0077-9
    1. Non-insulin-dependent diabetes—Diet therapy—Recipes.
2. Desserts.    I. Title.    II. Title: Type 2 diabetes desserts
cookbook.    III. Title: Type two diabetes desserts cookbook.
RC662.S642 1999
641.5'6314—dc21                                                99-26965
                                                                    CIP


Design by Kate Mueller


Published by Lowell House
A division of NTC/Contemporary Publishing Group, Inc.
4255 West Touhy Avenue, Lincolnwood
(Chicago), Illinois 60646-1975 U.S.A.

Printed in the United States of America
International Standard Book Number: 0-7373-0077-9
99 00 01 02 03 04 RRD 18 17 16 15 14 13 12 11 10 9 8 7 6 5 4 3 2 1

I dedicate this book to my daughters, Ruth Soneral and Janice Soneral Sutula, for their love, encouragement, and support. With all of the progress being made in diabetes research and education, there is a possibility that they will see a world without diabetes.

# CONTENTS

# CONTENTS

# FOREWORD

When I heard that Lois had been asked to write another diabetic cookbook, I asked her if she had enough recipes for another book. That was a silly question. The real question was which recipes to leave out.

Over the years, Lois has collected hundreds of recipes. I understand many are passed down through her family, and she has picked up many from friends. The majority of the recipes existed prior to her developing diabetes and, therefore, often have high fat and carbohydrate content. I have asked her what the process is in developing her new recipes, and found out that it is not as simple as cutting down on the fat and sugar content. Doing that would have led to something much less than the original product. Lois takes one of her original recipes, adjusts the ingredients, and tests her results. She may make multiple versions of the same basic recipe, which not only makes it diabetically correct, but true to the original flavor. In fact, our office had the pleasure of participating in her "recipe development" earlier this year. She brought our office several of her desserts for critique by our staff, and they were all a big hit!

Due to the success of her first cookbook, *The Type II Diabetes Cookbook,* Lois has been very active in traveling, working on new recipes, and participating in diabetic education in various places. Again, I can highly recommend her new cookbook, not only for Type 2 diabetics, but also for people who are generally interested in cutting down on fat content as well.

CHARLES L. CHAVEZ, M.D.

# ACKNOWLEDGMENTS

To my family for their patience, caring, and support as well as for eating the recipes that I have created. Special thanks to:

My daughter, Ruth Soneral, for being my computer guru and eagle-eyed proofreader, and for all of the time and effort she contributed to making this book a reality.

My daughter, Janice Soneral Sutula, for her word-processing expertise, all of the time and energy she has spent learning about diabetes, and for loaning her kitchen to me for recipe R&D when I winter in New Mexico.

My husband, Carl Soneral, for eating all the recipe experiments, telling me which dishes he likes, and taking me out to eat when he doesn't like them.

My son-in-law, Ronald Sutula, for encouraging me to try new recipes, being willing to eat them, and giving me "his arm to lean on."

Charles L. Chavez, M.D., for writing the foreword for this second book, as well as the first. He knows more about my diabetes than anyone else and talks with me and listens to me. Without him, I would not be alive and well.

Lowell House and especially Maria Magallanes, managing editor, and Bud Sperry, associate publisher, for diligently working with me on this book.

Beverly J. Spears, R.D., C.D.E., L.D., who taught me so much about nutrition, for writing an endorsement again, giving permission to use the 50/50 plate and nutritional management program that she created, and being my friend.

Dottie Gorzynski, B.S.N./R.N., my mentor and friend, for another endorsement, taste-testing recipes, proofreading, and providing a lot of encouragement.

Alan Mast, D.P.M., for taking excellent care of my feet when I am in Michigan, writing an endorsement for this book, and giving permission to use his materials.

Gerard Kerbleski, D.P.M., for writing an endorsement for this book and taking excellent care of my feet when I am in New Mexico.

Mark Plamp, R.Ph., for writing an endorsement for this book.

Susan Sommerfeldt, mother of a juvenile diabetic, Samantha, for her family's taste-testing foods, helping with research and development of this book, and writing an endorsement.

Sherrie and Rudy Simek, for taste-testing foods and writing an endorsement for this book.

Jacky Jeter, for her encouragement, use of her computer and printer when Ruth's got hit by lightning, taste-testing recipes, and writing an endorsement for this book.

Phyllis Young, Jeanette and George Petersen, Helen and Arnold Nelson, Carolyn Witter, Guy and Nancy Merskin, Rosemary Hansen, Chuck and Jeanne Andersen High, and Judy Hauser, for all their help with feedback on recipes, proofreading, and general support in making this book happen.

My diabetes support groups in Michigan and New Mexico, for sharing thoughts and feelings with me.

Memorial Medical Center of West Michigan for permission to reprint their materials.

The American Diabetes Association.

My Write People group, for sharing writing skills, listening to me, participating in taste-testing recipes for the research and development, and for your "feedback."

My relatives, friends, and all the terrific positive people I have met along this incredible journey, for all of the encouragement that you have given me.

To God, "for keeping His arm around my shoulder." He has given me the guidance, strength, determination, courage, and knowledge to control my diabetes. Along with this, my faith, love, and patience have increased.

Finally, thanks to the more than a hundred people who attended the R&D luncheons and suppers for giving me excellent feedback.

# INTRODUCTION

I am a diabetic! When I was diagnosed with Type 2 diabetes in March 1991, I needed recipes to get my diabetes under control. When I could not find ones that I wanted, I wrote a cookbook, *The Type II Diabetes Cookbook*.

Diabetes is a genetic disease and a metabolic disorder that affects the way food is converted into energy by the body. The onset of Type 2 diabetes usually occurs in midlife. The pancreas still produces insulin, but the body cells cannot make use of the insulin as it should. In Type 1 diabetes, which frequently begins in childhood, the pancreas makes no insulin so it has to be injected into the body. While most Type 1 diabetics are of normal weight, Type 2s are usually overweight.

Diabetes does not have to be an end to normal living, but rather it can be a beginning to a healthier, happier life. By taking care of your diabetes, you can give your life a new meaning. Lowering your cholesterol to more than 300 mg per day, eating right, and exercising, will be beneficial to your health (see Appendix B).

Dr. Charles L. Chavez of Albuquerque, New Mexico, told me that he would teach me what to do. He sent me to LaVerne Hohnstreiter, R.N., C.D.E., at the Diabetes Center in Albuquerque, New Mexico. She and Beverly Spears R.N., C.D.E., L.D., R.D., taught me how to control my diabetes, my blood glucose readings, and my diet. They also started me on an exercise regimen, and with Dr. Chavez's expertise, I learned how to control my diabetes.

Following certain guidelines can help you achieve that goal:

1. *Monitor your blood glucose readings every day.* Self-monitoring makes your diabetes more manageable.

2. *Exercise regularly.* Do any exercises that appeal to you, but do them every day. Cross-train: do more than one type of exercise, both for the psychological advantage of variety and to exercise different muscles. Exercise burns calories, builds lean tissue (muscle), and increases your basal metabolic rate, not only when you are exercising, but also when you are at rest.

3. *Join a support group.* Learn from others about their coping skills, concerns, feelings, problems, and successes. And share yours with others.

4. *Read food labels.* If sugar is listed as one of the first three ingredients, do not buy the product as there is a lot of sugar in it. (*Note:* an exception is angel food cake.) Diabetics want to avoid foods that contain a lot of sugar. Learn to recognize other words for sugar, such as corn syrup, dextrose, honey, fructose, maple syrup, and sorghum.

5. *Learn about your medications and insulin from your doctor.* Work with your doctor and other health care providers, including your certified diabetes educator, nutritionist, and dietitian. *You are a part of that team!*

6. *Do not feel overwhelmed by all you need to know.* Ask for information about your diabetes to become confident about your health and yourself.

7. *Change your eating habits.* Follow your diet. Take a positive step toward a healthier lifestyle. Eating correctly will make you feel better, look better, and also reduce the risk of a variety of health problems. A diet that is good for diabetics is good for everyone. You do not have to sacrifice taste, satisfaction, or the company of other diners. The recipes in this book are delicious and can be enjoyed by all and can taste good too.

I decided to write the first cookbook to provide diabetics good, wholesome foods that are not only low in sugar but also low in fat and cholesterol. We need recipes that are traditional, delicious, and that include easily obtained ingredients. I have found that it is easier to follow my diet when I include some favorite recipes that I have modified. I have also included new ones that I have developed.

Using these guidelines, I achieved my goal of getting off insulin by May 1992. After six years of being off *all* medications for my diabetes, I have the wonderful "side-effects" of feeling great, looking good, and avoiding the complications of diabetes. I will keep doing whatever it takes to maintain my good health and be the best controlled diabetic that I can be.

Many of these recipes contain a small amount of sugar. Sugar adds more than sweetness, it also adds bulk, which is necessary for a baked product to rise and to be light, tender, and delicious. Along with fat modification, it makes a better tasting and textured product. There are excellent sugar substitutes on the market that can be used as well (see Appendix D).

There was a wonderful response to my first book. I first told my family and friends, "This book will not change my life." Wrong! That was when the fun began. I had requests for book signings at book stores from Traverse City to Muskegon, Michigan, and in other states. Area newspaper reporters and radio talk show hosts interviewed me with questions about diabetes, nutrition, and "how to do it all." I was asked to speak at health fairs and similar engagements. Area restaurants and tea rooms had special luncheons using my recipes, and I have also spoken to several diabetes groups, including the quarterly meeting of the New Mexico Certified Diabetes Educators in Albuquerque, New Mexico, in February 1998. They told me that I was a diabetes professional's dream because I did all the things that they tell their patients to do, and then "I took the ball, ran with it, and really scored." Perhaps people are attracted by personal experience in finding diabetic control or the chance to transform old favorite recipes into acceptable dietary levels.

Whatever the reason, the first book has been very popular and generated a demand for more recipes. Desserts are the foods that are not adequately addressed in most other diabetic cookbooks and are clearly what diabetics want. I have heard so often that diabetics cannot have desserts or that they will never be able to have pie again. My response was, "Why not?" These foods, modified for the needs of diabetics, will make us less inclined to cheat on our diets.

As I began to work on my second book, I decided to involve many people in tasting the recipes. I have had several "research and development" (R&D) luncheons and suppers, both in Michigan and in New Mexico, where I usually served a beverage, breads, salads, and desserts. I have also taken breads and cookies to local offices and meetings for coffee breaks. Every recipe in this book has been "tongue-tested" by over one hundred people, and the response was heartwarming. Recipes were voted on for appearance, taste, and texture. Some of the comments from guests included, "You can cook for me anytime"; "If you have another luncheon I'd like to be invited"; "We are looking forward to the book being published"; "It's a 10 on a scale of 1 to 10"; "I can't believe that this is a diabetic recipe"; "The best place in town to eat is at your house"; and "Delicious!" I am grateful for the excellent feedback from people who attended these get-togethers and taste-tested the food.

My experience is that when you crave a special food, go ahead and have it. If you substitute something else, you will still crave that special food. So eat it. Resume your diet the next day and do not feel guilty. At one of the meetings where I spoke, Bill, a young man newly diagnosed with Type 2 diabetes, was angry, upset, and in denial of his illness. He said that what he wanted to do was to go out and have a hot fudge sundae. I told him to go ahead and do that as he would continue craving it and nothing else would take its place. He responded, "You're not listening." I said that yes I was listening, but go ahead and have it and resume your diet the next day. I talked with him two weeks later after he had had the hot fudge sundae. He said he couldn't even finish all of it because "it was too rich and too sweet," although he had eaten all of his ice cream. He said that after that he did not want another hot fudge sundae ever again.

A diabetic can lead a healthier and fuller lifestyle. Diabetes has certainly not slowed me down. In fact, diabetes and the changes I have made as a result have opened my life and given it new meaning.

# COOKIES

## General Baking Hints

- If brown sugar is hard, grate with a cheese grater.
- Dip a spoon into a cup of hot water before measuring solid shortening and it will slip off easily without sticking to the spoon.
- Fresh egg shells are rough and chalky, and old eggs are smooth and shiny.
- If you have oversweetened a dish, add a dash of salt.
- Lumpy sugar will not be lumpy if you place it in the refrigerator for 24 to 30 hours.
- To remove food that is stuck in a casserole, fill the pan with boiling water and 2 tablespoons of baking soda and let stand for a few minutes.
- Use a toothbrush to clean cheese, onion, lemon peel, or egg out of grater before washing it.
- Apply baking soda to spills on your stove top and burner rings. Then rub with a damp cloth, rinse with clear water, and dry well.

# Almond-Topped Cookies

    ½ cup low-fat margarine

    ¼ cup sugar

    6 packets Acesulfame K sugar substitute

    ½ cup non-fat cream cheese

    2 teaspoons vanilla extract

    ½ teaspoon almond extract

    1 teaspoon baking powder

    2 cups all-purpose flour

    20 blanched almonds, halved

1. Preheat oven to 375°. Grease baking sheets with margarine.
2. Melt the margarine in microwave until lightly browned. Let cool and place in a medium bowl. Add the sugar, sugar substitute, and cream cheese. Using an electric mixer, beat until smooth and well blended. Add the vanilla and almond extracts and baking powder. Mix well. Add the flour and mix until the dough is crumbly. Chill for at least 1 hour.
3. Using your hands, roll the dough into walnut-size balls, and place on a greased baking sheet. Press ½ almond into the top of each cookie.
4. Bake for 10 to 12 minutes, or until lightly browned.

YIELD: 40 COOKIES     0.5 G FAT     12 MG SODIUM
SERVING SIZE: 1 COOKIE     TRACE FIBER     TRACE CHOLESTEROL
CALORIES: 51

# Coconut Cookies

 1 tablespoon low-fat margarine

1³/₄ cups all-purpose flour

 1 cup flaked coconut

 ¹/₃ cup sugar

   Acesulfame K sugar substitute
   equivalent to ¹/₃ cup sugar

 ¹/₂ teaspoon baking soda

 ¹/₄ teaspoon salt

 ¹/₂ cup low-fat margarine

 1 large egg

 ¹/₄ cup water

 2 teaspoons coconut flavoring

1. Preheat oven to 375°. Grease baking sheets.
2. In a large mixing bowl combine the flour, coconut, sugar, sugar substitute, baking soda, and salt. Mix until well blended. Add the margarine, egg, water, and flavoring. Using an electric mixer at medium speed, beat until well blended. Drop by teaspoonfuls onto baking sheets.
3. Bake for 10 minutes, or until cookies are lightly browned on the bottom. Remove and cool at room temperature.

YIELD: 48 COOKIES        5 G FAT              TRACE SODIUM
SERVING SIZE: 2 COOKIES  1 G PROTEIN          11 MG CHOLESTEROL
CALORIES: 101            13 G CARBOHYDRATES

# Applesauce Cookies

1 cup all-purpose flour

1 teaspoon baking soda

1 teaspoon cinnamon

¼ teaspoon salt

¼ teaspoon cloves

¼ teaspoon nutmeg

½ cup unsweetened applesauce

¼ cup vegetable oil

Acesulfame K sugar substitute equivalent to 1 teaspoon sugar

1. Preheat oven to 375°.
2. Sift together the flour, baking soda, cinnamon, salt, cloves, and nutmeg. In a medium bowl, combine the applesauce, oil, and sugar substitute. Add the applesauce mixture to the flour mixture and mix well. Drop by rounded teaspoonfuls onto ungreased baking sheets.
3. Bake for 12 to 15 minutes, or until firm.

YIELD: 24 COOKIES  
SERVING SIZE: 1 COOKIE  
CALORIES: 42

2 G FAT  
0.5 G PROTEIN  
2.4 G CARBOHYDRATES

# Ginger-Molasses Cookies

*Because they contain no dairy products, these quick treats
are also suitable for people on a lactose-free diet.*

non-stick vegetable cooking spray

¹/₄ cup sugar

Acesulfame K sugar substitute
equivalent to ¹/₄ cup sugar

¹/₂ cup hot water

¹/₂ cup molasses

¹/₄ cup shortening

1 egg

2 cups all-purpose flour

1 teaspoon baking soda

¹/₂ teaspoon salt

³/₄ teaspoon ground ginger

¹/₂ teaspoon cinnamon

¹/₂ teaspoon nutmeg

¹/₂ teaspoon cloves

1. Preheat oven to 375°. Coat baking sheets with non-stick
   cooking spray.
2. In a large bowl, combine the sugar, sugar substitute, hot
   water, molasses, shortening, and egg. Add the flour, baking
   soda, salt, ginger, cinnamon, nutmeg, and cloves. Mix well.
   Drop by rounded teaspoonfuls onto baking sheets.
3. Bake for 10 to 15 minutes, or until brown. Remove from pans
   to cool.

YIELD: 40 COOKIES | 2 G FAT | 40 MG SODIUM
SERVING SIZE: 1 COOKIE | 0.5 G PROTEIN | 30 MG POTASSIUM
CALORIES: 50 | 10 G CARBOHYDRATES |

# Crunchy Cereal Cookies

¼ cup vegetable oil

¼ cup sugar

¼ cup brown sugar

Acesulfame K sugar substitute equivalent to ⅛ cup sugar

brown sugar substitute equivalent to ⅛ cup brown sugar

1 egg

1 teaspoon vanilla extract

1 cup all-purpose flour

½ teaspoon baking powder

½ teaspoon baking soda

¼ teaspoon salt

1 cup Rice Krispies™ cereal

1 cup quick oatmeal

½ cup flaked coconut

1. Preheat oven to 375°.
2. In a large bowl, beat together the oil, sugars, sugar substitutes, egg, and vanilla. In a medium bowl, mix together the flour, baking powder, baking soda, and salt. Add the flour mixture to the oil mixture. Mix well. Add the cereal, oatmeal, and coconut and mix well. Using your hands, roll the dough into balls 1 inch in diameter. Place on ungreased baking sheets.
3. Bake for 10 to 12 minutes, or until firm.

YIELD: 30 COOKIES      3.3 G FAT
SERVING SIZE: 1 COOKIE      15 MG CARBOHYDRATES
CALORIES: 95
EXCHANGES: 1 STARCH/BREAD

# Coconut Cherry Drop Cookies

non-stick vegetable cooking spray

1 1/4 cups all-purpose flour

1/4 cup sugar

Acesulfame K sugar substitute equivalent to 1/4 cup sugar

1/2 teaspoon salt

1 teaspoon baking powder

1/2 cup low-fat margarine, softened

1 teaspoon almond extract

1 egg

1 cup flaked coconut

1/2 cup chopped pecans or walnuts

1/4 cup chopped maraschino cherries, drained

1. Preheat oven to 375°. Coat baking sheets with non-stick cooking spray.
2. In a large bowl, combine the flour, sugar, sugar substitute, salt, baking powder, margarine, extract, and egg. Mix well. Stir in the coconut, nuts, and cherries. Using your hands, shape dough into small balls, 1/2 to 3/4 inch in diameter. Place on baking sheets.
3. Bake for 10 to 12 minutes, or until lightly browned around the edges.

YIELD: 48 COOKIES
SERVING SIZE: 1 COOKIE
CALORIES: 64 EACH

8 G FAT
2 G PROTEIN
12 G CARBOHYDRATES

105 MG SODIUM
55 MG POTASSIUM

# Pecan Cookies

*Easy to make and a delicious snack,*
*store these nutty cookies in the freezer.*

1 tablespoon low-fat margarine

2 large egg whites

$1/4$ teaspoon cream of tartar

brown sugar substitute
equivalent to $1/2$ cup brown sugar

$1/4$ cup brown sugar

1 teaspoon vanilla extract

1 cup chopped pecans

$1 1/2$ cups corn flakes

1. Preheat oven to 250°. Grease baking sheets.
2. In a large bowl, using an electric mixer at high speed, beat the egg whites and cream of tartar until stiff and firm peaks hold. Add the brown sugar substitute and brown sugar and continue beating to form a meringue. Stir in the vanilla extract, pecans, and corn flakes. Mix well. Drop by table-spoonfuls onto baking sheets.
3. Bake for 30 to 35 minutes, or until firm.
4. Store in a covered container in the freezer. If stored at room temperature they become soft. (Do not refrigerate.) Remove from freezer to thaw for 5 minutes before serving.

YIELD: 30 COOKIES    2.4 G FAT    0 MG CHOLESTEROL
SERVING SIZE: 1 COOKIE    0.5 G PROTEIN
CALORIES: 69    11 G CARBOHYDRATES

# Crescent Roll Cookies

❧

non-stick vegetable cooking spray

1 8-ounce can crescent rolls

1 egg

$\frac{1}{2}$ cup chopped pecans or walnuts

$\frac{1}{4}$ cup sugar

$\frac{1}{4}$ cup light corn syrup

Acesulfame K sugar substitute equivalent to $\frac{1}{2}$ cup sugar

1 tablespoon low-fat margarine, melted

1 teaspoon vanilla extract

1. Preheat oven to 375°. Coat a 9-by-13-inch pan with non-stick cooking spray.
2. Unroll crescent rolls into 2 rectangles. Place in pan and press over bottom and up the sides to form a crust. Bake for 5 minutes.
3. In a medium bowl, combine the egg, nuts, sugar, corn syrup, sugar substitute, margarine, and vanilla extract. Pour over the crust.
4. Bake for 20 minutes. Cool and cut into bars.

YIELD: 36 BARS
SERVING SIZE: 2 INCHES
    BY 1 $\frac{1}{2}$ INCHES
CALORIES: 62

2.5 G FAT
0.5 G PROTEIN
9 G CARBOHYDRATES

85 MG SODIUM

# Chocolate Nut Refrigerator Cookies

½ cup sugar

Acesulfame K sugar substitute
equivalent to ½ cup sugar

¾ cup low-fat margarine, softened

2 ounces unsweetened chocolate, melted

1 teaspoon vanilla extract

1 egg

2¼ cups all-purpose flour

¼ teaspoon salt

½ teaspoon baking soda

½ teaspoon cinnamon

½ cup chopped walnuts

1. In a large bowl, combine the sugar, sugar substitute, margarine, chocolate, vanilla extract, and egg. Mix well. Stir in the flour, salt, baking soda, cinnamon, and walnuts. Mix until well blended. Divide dough in half and shape each into a roll 2 inches in diameter. Wrap in waxed paper and refrigerate for 3½ to 4 hours, or until firm.

2. Preheat oven to 400°.

3. Cut each roll into 36 slices and place on ungreased baking sheets.

4. Bake for 8 to 10 minutes, or until lightly browned. Do not overbake. Remove from baking sheet immediately and place on waxed paper to cool.

YIELD: 72 COOKIES    6 G FAT    70 MG SODIUM
SERVING SIZE: 1 COOKIE    1 G PROTEIN    30 MG POTASSIUM
CALORIES: 53    12 G CARBOHYDRATES

# Christmas Cutout Cookies

½ cup shortening

Acesulfame K  sugar substitute
equivalent to 3 tablespoons sugar

1 egg

2¾ cups all-purpose flour; set aside ¼ cup

2 teaspoons baking powder

½ teaspoon salt

½ cup 2% milk

2 tablespoons water

1 teaspoon vanilla extract

1. In a medium bowl, cream the shortening. Add the sugar substitute and egg and beat well. In another medium bowl, sift together 2½ cups of the flour, the baking powder, and salt. In a measuring cup, combine milk, water, and vanilla extract. Alternately stir the flour mixture and pour the milk mixture into the creamed mixture, mixing well after each addition. Refrigerate for 1 hour.

2. Preheat oven to 350°. Grease baking sheets with margarine (shortening). Sprinkle remaining ¼ cup flour on work surface as needed.

3. Roll out the dough to ¹⁄₁₆-inch thick and cut with cookie cutter. Place on baking sheets.

4. Bake for 8 minutes, or until lightly browned. Remove from oven and place on rack to cool.

   *Note:* Decorations will add to the nutritional content.

YIELD: 100 2-INCH COOKIES          CALORIES: 58
SERVING SIZE: 3 COOKIES            EXCHANGES: ⅔ STARCH/BREAD

# Sugar-Free Orange Cookies

½ cup low-fat margarine, softened

1 egg

1 tablespoon grated orange peel

½ cup unsweetened orange juice

2 cups all-purpose flour

2 teaspoons baking powder

½ teaspoon cinnamon

½ teaspoon salt

½ cup mashed banana

½ cup chopped pecans

1. Preheat oven to 375°.
2. In a large bowl, stir together the margarine and egg. Add the orange peel and orange juice. Mix well. In a medium bowl, stir together the flour, baking powder, cinnamon, and salt. Add the flour mixture and banana to the margarine mixture and stir until well blended. Stir in the nuts. Drop dough by teaspoonfuls onto ungreased baking sheets.
3. Bake for 15 to 20 minutes, or until lightly browned.

YIELD: 24 COOKIES
SERVING SIZE: 1 COOKIE
CALORIES: 80
EXCHANGES: 1½ FAT; 1 FRUIT; 1 STARCH/BREAD

# Sugar-Free Apple Cookies

½ cup low-fat margarine, softened

1 egg

1 tablespoon unsweetened applesauce

½ cup unsweetened apple juice

½ cup mashed banana

2 cups all-purpose flour

2 teaspoons baking powder

½ teaspoon cinnamon

½ teaspoon nutmeg

½ teaspoon salt

½ cup chopped walnuts

1. Preheat oven to 375°.
2. In a large bowl, stir together the margarine and egg. Add the applesauce, apple juice, and banana. Mix well. In a medium bowl, stir together the flour, baking powder, cinnamon, nutmeg, and salt. Add the flour mixture to the margarine mixture and stir until well blended. Stir in the nuts. Drop by teaspoonfuls onto ungreased baking sheets.
3. Bake for 15 to 20 minutes, or until lightly browned.

YIELD: 24 COOKIES
SERVING SIZE: 1 COOKIE
CALORIES: 80
EXCHANGES: 1½ FAT; ¼ FRUIT; 1 STARCH/BREAD

# Sugar-Free Peanut Butter Cookies

1 1/2 cups all-purpose flour

1 1/2 teaspoons baking powder

1/2 teaspoon salt

1/4 cup low-fat margarine

1/2 cup lite creamy peanut butter

1/2 teaspoon grated orange peel

1 1/2 teaspoons vanilla extract

1 egg, well beaten

1/3 cup unsweetened orange juice

Acesulfame K sugar substitute
equivalent to 1/2 cup sugar

1. Preheat oven to 400°.
2. Into a medium bowl, sift together the flour, baking powder, and salt. In a large bowl, cream together the margarine, peanut butter, orange peel, and vanilla extract. Add the egg, orange juice, and sugar substitute. Blend well. Gradually add the flour mixture, stirring well after each addition. Using your hands, roll 1 tablespoon dough to form balls. Place on ungreased baking sheet, flatten with a fork.
3. Bake for 15 minutes, or until lightly browned.

YIELD: 48
SERVING SIZE: 2 COOKIES
CALORIES: 190
EXCHANGES: 2 FAT; 1/2 STARCH/BREAD

# Coconut Macaroons

*Always a favorite cookie!*

¹/₂ teaspoon low-fat margarine

¹/₂ cup all-purpose flour

2 cups flaked coconut

¹/₂ cup egg whites, at room temperature

¹/₂ teaspoon cream of tartar

1 cup powdered sugar

1 teaspoon coconut flavoring

1. Preheat oven to 325°. Grease baking sheets with margarine.
2. In a medium bowl, combine the flour and coconut together. In a large bowl, using an electric mixture at high speed, beat the egg whites and cream of tartar until stiff. Add the powdered sugar and coconut flavoring and beat together. Gradually add the flour mixture, stirring after each addition. Drop by tablespoonfuls onto baking sheets.
3. Bake for 25 minutes, or until firm and lightly browned. Store in a covered container in the freezer or in a loosely covered container at room temperature.

YIELD: 20 MACAROONS          3 G FAT
SERVING SIZE: 1 MACAROON     1 G PROTEIN
CALORIES: 62                 9 G CARBOHYDRATES

# Coconut Pecan Macaroons

*This simple cookie needs few ingredients. It is easy to make with less calories than classic pecan macaroons.*

non-stick vegetable cooking spray
²/₃ cup non-fat sweetened condensed milk
3 cups finely shredded or flaked coconut
1 teaspoon vanilla extract
¹/₂ cup chopped pecans

1. Preheat oven to 350°. Coat baking sheets with non-stick cooking spray.
2. In a bowl, combine the condensed milk, coconut, and vanilla extract. Stir in the pecans. Blend well. Drop by teaspoonfuls onto baking sheets.
3. Bake for 8 to 10 minutes, or until lightly browned. Remove from baking sheet immediately. Store in a tightly covered container.

YIELD: 90 COOKIES          1 G FAT                    9 MG SODIUM
SERVING SIZE: 1 COOKIE     2 G CARBOHYDRATES          1 MG CHOLESTEROL
CALORIES: 48

# BARS

## Tips for Baking Bars and Cookies

- When baking bars and cookies, be sure to follow directions on pan preparation. It does make a difference.
- Use a good cookie sheet. Place dough on a cooled sheet as dough spreads on a warm one.
- To brown cookies or bars evenly, use a bright shiny pan or line with aluminum foil.
- Cool bars and cookies completely before placing in storage containers.
- Some cookies tend to harden. To keep them moist, place a slice of bread in the cookie jar.
- To save time, work with three or four sheets that you can fill and bake.
- Bars and cookies can be frozen for up to two to six months. Arrange them in a tin lined with aluminum foil and separate layers with foil. Thaw cookies by placing them on a plate and allowing them to stand for 15 to 20 minutes.

# Chocolate Drizzle Bars

½ cup low-fat margarine

½ cup unsweetened orange juice

1 egg

2 cups all-purpose flour

Acesulfame K sugar substitute
equivalent to ¼ cup sugar

2 teaspoons baking powder

½ teaspoon salt

2 teaspoons vanilla extract

½ cup chopped walnuts

1 ounce unsweetened chocolate

1. Preheat oven to 375°. Grease a 9-by-13-inch baking pan with margarine.
2. In a large bowl, using an electric mixer at medium speed, beat the margarine, orange juice, and egg. Add the flour, sugar substitute, baking powder, and salt. Blend well. Add the vanilla extract and walnuts and blend well again. The dough will be stiff. Spread evenly in prepared pan.
3. Bake approximately 20 minutes, or until lightly browned around the edges.
4. Meanwhile, melt the unsweetened chocolate in microwave. Drizzle chocolate over uncut baked bars. Store cooled bars in a tightly covered container. These bars will freeze well.

YIELD: 48 BARS
SERVING SIZE: 2 BARS, 1 INCH BY 1 INCH
CALORIES: 50 PER BAR
EXCHANGES: 1 FAT; ½ STARCH/BREAD

# Pumpkin Bars

❧

*The hardest part of making these favorites is waiting
for them to cool! These may be made ahead and frozen
for up to 6 weeks, making them an ideal choice for a
holiday party. Thaw for at least 20 minutes before serving.*

$\frac{1}{2}$ teaspoon low-fat margarine

3 large eggs

$\frac{1}{3}$ scant cup granulated sugar

brown sugar substitute equivalent
to $\frac{1}{3}$ cup brown sugar

$\frac{1}{2}$ cup vegetable oil

16 ounces canned solid-pack pumpkin

2 cups all-purpose flour

2 teaspoons baking powder

1 teaspoon baking soda

$\frac{1}{2}$ teaspoon salt

$1\frac{1}{2}$ teaspoons cinnamon

$\frac{1}{2}$ teaspoon nutmeg

$\frac{1}{2}$ teaspoon cloves

$\frac{1}{4}$ teaspoon ginger

1. Preheat oven to 350°. Grease a 9-by-13-inch pan.
2. In a large bowl, using an electric mixer at medium speed, beat the eggs, sugar, sugar substitute, oil, and pumpkin until smooth. Stir in the flour, baking powder, baking soda,

and salt. Blend well. Add the cinnamon, nutmeg, cloves, and ginger and blend well again. Pour into prepared pan.
3. Bake for 25 to 30 minutes, or until a tester inserted in the center comes out clean. Cool and cut into 2¼-by-2-inch pieces.

YIELD: 24 SERVINGS
SERVING SIZE: 2¼ INCHES
   BY 2 INCHES
CALORIES: 106

4 G FAT
2 G PROTEIN
30 MG CHOLESTEROL
12 G CARBOHYDRATES

110 MG SODIUM

# Lemon Pie Bars

*Great, refreshing citrus taste.*

CRUST:  ³/4 cup low-fat margarine, softened

¹/3 cup confectioners' sugar

1 ¹/4 cups all-purpose flour

FILLING:  4 eggs

¹/2 cup sugar

Acesulfame K sugar substitute equivalent to ¹/3 cup sugar

¹/2 cup lemon juice

¹/3 cup all-purpose flour

¹/2 teaspoon baking powder

8 ounces non-fat lemon yogurt

1. Preheat oven to 350°.
2. Combine the crust ingredients until mixture is crumbly. Press into bottom of a 9-by-13-inch pan. Bake 20 minutes, or until golden brown.
3. Meanwhile, in a large bowl using an electric mixer at medium speed, beat the eggs until thickened. Gradually add the sugar, sugar substitute, lemon juice, flour, and baking powder. Blend well. Gently stir in the yogurt. Pour mixture into hot crust.
4. Bake for 20 minutes, or until a tester inserted in the center comes out clean.

YIELD: 20 SERVINGS
SERVING SIZE: 2¹/4 INCHES
   BY 2¹/2 INCHES
CALORIES: 70

2.5 G FAT
2.5 G PROTEIN
43 MG CHOLESTEROL
4 G CARBOHYDRATES

24 MG SODIUM

# Pecan Pie Bars

*Their super taste makes these a
favorite for those with a "sweet tooth."*

1 ⅓ cups all-purpose flour

¼ cup plus 2 tablespoons brown sugar

½ cup low-fat margarine

brown sugar substitute
equivalent to ¼ cup brown sugar

2 eggs

½ cup light corn syrup

½ cup finely chopped pecans

2 tablespoons low-fat margarine, melted

1 teaspoon vanilla extract

⅛ teaspoon salt

1. Preheat oven to 350°.
2. In a small bowl, mix the flour and 2 tablespoons brown sugar. Using your fingers, work in the ½ cup margarine until the dough begins to hold together. Press into the bottom of a 9-inch square pan. Bake for 12 to 15 minutes, or until firm.
3. In a medium bowl, lightly beat ¼ cup brown sugar, brown sugar substitute, and eggs. Add the corn syrup, pecans, 2 tablespoons margarine, vanilla, and salt. Mix well. Pour over the baked crust.
4. Bake for 25 minutes, or until the edges are lightly browned. Cool in the pan.

YIELD: 27 BARS       3 G FAT       18 MG SODIUM
SERVING SIZE: 1 INCH BY 3 INCHES   0.5 G PROTEIN
CALORIES: 85       4.5 G CARBOHYDRATES

# Low-Fat Chocolate Brownies

non-stick vegetable cooking spray

³/₄ cup semisweet chocolate chips

1 14-ounce can non-fat sweetened condensed milk

¹/₄ cup unsweetened cocoa

3 egg whites

¹/₃ cup all-purpose flour

1 teaspoon baking powder

1 teaspoon vanilla extract

1. Preheat oven to 350°. Coat a 9-by-13-inch pan with non-stick cooking spray.
2. In a medium saucepan over low heat, melt the chocolate chips with the condensed milk and cocoa. Cool for 15 minutes, then add the egg whites, flour, baking powder, and vanilla extract. Blend well. Pour into the prepared pan.
3. Bake for 20 to 25 minutes, or until a tester inserted in the center comes out clean. Cool in the pan. Store tightly covered at room temperature.

YIELD: 20 BROWNIES    2 G FAT      45 MG SODIUM
SERVING SIZE: 2¹/₄ INCHES   3 G PROTEIN    50 MG CHOLESTEROL
    BY 2¹/₂ INCHES    18 G CARBOHYDRATES
CALORIES: 110

# Butterscotch Blondies

❧

*All the blondie variations are a fabulous*
*snack that was popular with all my taste-testers.*

non-stick vegetable cooking spray
2¼ cups all-purpose flour
2½ teaspoons baking powder
½ teaspoon salt
½ cup brown sugar
brown sugar substitute
equivalent to ½ cup brown sugar
⅓ cup low-fat margarine
2 eggs
1 teaspoon vanilla extract
½ cup water
12 ounces butterscotch chips
¼ cup crushed pecans

1. Preheat oven to 350°. Coat a 9-by-13-inch pan with non-stick cooking spray.
2. In a small bowl, combine the flour, baking powder, and salt. In a large bowl, combine the sugar, sugar substitute, margarine, eggs, and vanilla extract. Mix until smooth. Gradually add the flour mixture alternately with the water to the sugar mixture, stirring well after each addition. Stir in the chips and nuts. The batter will be stiff. Spread into the prepared pan.
3. Bake for 20 to 25 minutes, or until golden brown. Cool in the pan.

YIELD: 48 PIECES    3.7 G FAT           70 MG SODIUM
SERVING SIZE: 1½ INCHES  1 G PROTEIN        0 MG CHOLESTEROL
    BY 1½ INCHES   16 G CARBOHYDRATES
CALORIES: 102

# Chocolate Chip Blondies

non-stick vegetable cooking spray

2¼ cups all-purpose flour

2½ teaspoons baking powder

½ teaspoon salt

½ cup brown sugar

brown sugar substitute
equivalent to ½ cup brown sugar

½ cup low-fat margarine, softened

2 eggs

1½ teaspoons vanilla extract

⅓ cup water

12 ounces semisweet chocolate chips

¼ cup chopped walnuts

1. Preheat oven to 350°. Coat a 9-by-13-inch pan with non-stick cooking spray.
2. In a small bowl, combine the flour, baking powder, and salt. In a large bowl, combine the sugar, sugar substitute, margarine, eggs, and vanilla extract. Mix until smooth. Gradually add the flour mixture alternately with the water to the sugar mixture, stirring well after each addition. Stir in the chips and nuts. The batter will be stiff. Spread into the prepared pan.
3. Bake for 20 to 25 minutes, or until lightly browned. Cool in the pan.

YIELD: 48 PIECES    3.7 G FAT    70 MG SODIUM
SERVING SIZE: 1½ INCHES    1 G PROTEIN    0 MG CHOLESTEROL
   BY 1½ INCHES    16 G CARBOHYDRATES
CALORIES: 102

# Peanut Butter Blondies

*Take a batch of blondies to a potluck and
you're bound to go home with an empty tray!*

non-stick vegetable cooking spray

2¼ cups all-purpose flour

2½ teaspoons baking powder

¼ teaspoon salt

½ cup brown sugar

brown sugar substitute
equivalent to ½ cup brown sugar

5 tablespoons low-fat margarine

2 eggs

1 teaspoon vanilla extract

⅓ cup water

10 ounces peanut butter chips

½ cup chopped pecans

1. Preheat oven to 350°. Coat a 9-by-13-inch pan with non-stick cooking spray.
2. In a small bowl, combine the flour, baking powder, and salt. In a large bowl, combine the sugar, sugar substitute, margarine, eggs, and vanilla extract. Mix until smooth. Gradually add the flour mixture alternately with the water to the sugar mixture, stirring well after each addition. Add the chips and nuts. The batter will be stiff. Spread into the prepared pan.
3. Bake for 20 to 25 minutes, or until the top is lightly browned. Cool in the pan.

YIELD: 48 PIECES
SERVING SIZE: 1½ INCHES
　BY 1½ INCHES
CALORIES: 88

3.5 G FAT
1 G PROTEIN
15 G CARBOHYDRATES

66 MG SODIUM

# Chocolate Chip Bars

non-stick vegetable cooking spray

1/3 cup low-fat margarine, softened

2 tablespoons honey

1/3 cup 2% milk

1 egg

1/3 cup frozen unsweetened
orange juice concentrate, thawed

1 teaspoon vanilla extract

1 1/2 cups all-purpose flour

1 teaspoon baking soda

1/8 teaspoon salt

1/4 cup semisweet chocolate chips

1. Preheat oven to 350°. Coat an 8-inch square pan with non-stick cooking spray, then lightly flour the pan.
2. In a small bowl, combine the margarine, honey, milk, egg, juice concentrate, and vanilla extract. In a large bowl, combine the flour, baking soda, and salt. Add the margarine mixture to the flour mixture and mix well. Stir in the chocolate chips. Spread into the prepared pan.
3. Bake for 25 to 30 minutes, or until a tester inserted in the center comes out clean.

YIELD: 15 SERVINGS     5 G FAT     30 MG SODIUM
SERVING SIZE: 2 1/2 INCHES     2 G PROTEIN
    BY 1 1/2 INCHES     10 G CARBOHYDRATES
CALORIES: 100

# CAKES

## Typical Pans & Baking Dishes

**4-Cup Baking Dish:**
>   9-inch pie plate
>   8-by-1¼-inch cake pan
>   7½-by-3½-inch loaf pan

**6-Cup Baking Dish:**
>   8-inch layer cake pan
>   10-inch pie plate
>   8½-by-3½-inch loaf pan

**8-Cup Baking Dish:**
>   8-inch square pan
>   11-by-7½-inch baking pan
>   9-by-5-inch loaf pan

**10-Cup Baking Dish:**
>   9-inch square pan
>   11¾-by-7½-inch baking pan
>   15-by-10-inch jelly roll pan

**Larger Baking Dishes:**

$13\frac{1}{2}$-by-$8\frac{1}{2}$-by-2-inch = 12 cups

9-by-13-by-2-inch = 15 cups

14-by-$10\frac{1}{2}$-by-$2\frac{1}{2}$-inch = 19 cup roasting pan

**Melon Mold:**

7-by-$5\frac{1}{2}$-by-4-inch mold = 6 cups

**Ring Mold:**

$8\frac{1}{2}$-by-$2\frac{1}{4}$-inch mold = $4\frac{1}{2}$ cups

$9\frac{1}{4}$-by-$2\frac{3}{4}$-inch = 8 cups

**Tube Pans:**

9-by-$3\frac{1}{2}$-inch angel food cake = 12 cups

10-by-4-inch angel food cake = 15 cups

# Chocolate Chip Snack Cake

❧

½ cup vegetable oil
¼ cup honey
1 large egg
½ cup rolled oats
1 cup whole-wheat flour
1 tablespoon baking powder
½ cup semisweet chocolate chips
¾ cup non-fat milk

1. Preheat oven to 350°. Use oil to prepare pan.
2. In a large bowl, cream together the oil, honey, and egg. Add the oats, flour, baking powder, chocolate chips, and milk. Stir to blend thoroughly. Pour the batter into the prepared pan.
3. Bake for 30 to 35 minutes.

YIELD: 12 SERVINGS
SERVING SIZE: 2 INCHES
   BY 2½ INCHES
CALORIES: 207
EXCHANGES: 1 FAT; 1 FRUIT;
   1 STARCH/BREAD

8 G FAT
4 G PROTEIN

347 MG SODIUM
28 G CARBOHYDRATES

# Banana-Strawberry Layered Angel Food Cake

❧

*Angel food cake is a wonderfully fat-free food. Use a purchased cake or make one from a package or your favorite recipe. Then use this guide to turn it into something fabulous. Because it looks great and tastes sensational, this fruit-filled cake is ideal for a party.*

½ cup evaporated non-fat milk, chilled

1¼ cups fresh sliced or defrosted frozen strawberries, drained with juice reserved

1 envelope (1 tablespoon) Knox™ unflavored gelatin

¼ cup cold water

red food coloring (optional)

1 12-inch prepared angel food cake

2 ripe bananas, thinly sliced fresh strawberries for garnish (optional)

1. Pour the milk into ice cube tray and freeze until ice crystals begin to form around edges. Measure the reserved strawberry juice, adding water to juice to make one cup.

2. In a saucepan, combine the gelatin with ¼ cup water to soften. Wait one minute, then heat gently until gelatin dissolves. Stir in reserved juice mixture and refrigerate until cool.

3. In a medium bowl, using an electric mixer at medium speed, beat the chilled gelatin mixture with the semifrozen

milk until peaks form. If desired, add a few drops of food coloring. Fold in the berries.

4. Using a serrated knife, slice the cake horizontally into three layers. Frost the first layer with one-third of the strawberry mixture and top with half of the banana slices. Add the second cake layer. Frost with half of the remaining strawberry mixture and top with remaining banana slices. Add the third cake layer. Frost the top of the cake with the remaining strawberry mixture.

5. Chill thoroughly before serving. Garnish with a few fresh strawberries, if desired.

YIELD: 16 SERVINGS    0.2 G FAT         67.5 MG SODIUM
SERVING SIZE: 1/16 CAKE  3.6 G PROTEIN     0.3 MG CHOLESTEROL
CALORIES: 133        30.1 G CARBOHYDRATES

# Pineapple Carrot Cake

❧

*Many people like this variation of a carrot cake.*
*The pineapple adds an interesting texture and sweetness*
*that allows the cake to be served without frosting.*

non-stick vegetable cooking spray

1/2 cup margarine, softened

3 eggs

1 cup frozen unsweetened pineapple
juice concentrate, thawed

2 teaspoons vanilla extract

2 1/2 cups all-purpose flour

2 teaspoons baking powder

1 teaspoon baking soda

1 teaspoon nutmeg

1 teaspoon cinnamon

1/4 teaspoon salt

3 cups grated carrots

1. Preheat oven to 350°. Coat a 9-by-13 inch baking pan with non-stick cooking spray.
2. In a large bowl, beat the margarine until creamy. Add the eggs, juice concentrate, and vanilla extract. In a medium bowl, combine the flour, baking powder, baking soda, nutmeg, cinnamon, and salt. Gradually add the flour mixture to the margarine mixture, beating well. Stir in the carrots. Mix well. Spread batter in the baking pan.
3. Bake for 35 minutes, or until a tester inserted in the center comes out clean. Cool on a rack.

YIELD: 12 SERVINGS     12 G FAT     300 MG SODIUM
SERVING SIZE: 1/12 CAKE     5 G PROTEIN     60 MG CHOLESTEROL
CALORIES: 260     30 G CARBOHYDRATES

# Brownstone Front Cake

*This is a very old recipe that my mother used to make. A favorite of the family, it is a unique but delicious chocolate cake. Originally, it took a lot of sugar and shortening and was not acceptable for my diabetes diet. I worked on it and modified it, so that now it will fit into a diabetic meal plan.*

non-stick vegetable cooking spray

½ cup low-fat margarine, softened

½ cup sugar

6 packets Acesulfame K sugar substitute equivalent to ½ cup sugar

¾ scant cup cocoa

½ cup hot water

2 eggs

½ cup 2% milk

1 teaspoon vanilla extract

1 teaspoon baking soda

2 cups all-purpose flour

1. Preheat oven to 350°. Coat a 9-by-13-inch pan with non-stick cooking spray.
2. In a large bowl, cream the margarine, sugar, and sugar substitute. In a small bowl, dissolve the cocoa in the hot water. Add the cocoa mixture to the creamed mixture. Add the eggs and mix well. Stir in the milk, vanilla extract, and baking soda. Blend well. Gradually add flour, stirring after each addition. Mix well. Pour into prepared pan.
3. Bake for 30 to 35 minutes, or until a tester inserted in the center comes out clean.

YIELD: 32 PIECES
SERVING SIZE: 1½ INCHES BY 2 INCHES
CALORIES: 80

1 G FAT
0.5 G PROTEIN
3 G CARBOHYDRATES

50 MG SODIUM
TRACE CHOLESTEROL

# Pumpkin Roll

*While this is time-consuming to make,
it's a great dessert with a festive look.*

CAKE:
- ³/₄ cup all-purpose flour
- ¹/₄ cup sugar
- Acesulfame K sugar substitute equivalent to ¹/₄ cup sugar
- 1¹/₄ teaspoons baking powder
- 1 teaspoon pumpkin pie spice
- 1 teaspoon cinnamon
- ¹/₂ teaspoon nutmeg
- ²/₃ cup canned solid-pack pumpkin
- 3 eggs
- 5 tablespoons confectioners' sugar

FILLING:
- 1¹/₄ cups non-fat ricotta cheese
- ¹/₄ cup confectioners' sugar
- 1 teaspoon vanilla extract
- ¹/₂ teaspoon lemon juice

1. Preheat oven to 350°. Line a 15¹/₄-by-10¹/₄-inch jelly roll pan with parchment paper and fold up the sides so that the pan bottom and sides are lined.
2. In a medium bowl, combine the flour, sugar, sugar substitute, baking powder, pumpkin pie spice, cinnamon, and nutmeg, and stir to mix well. Add the pumpkin and eggs and blend until well mixed. Spread the batter evenly in the pan.

3. Bake for 10 to 12 minutes, or until the cake springs back when touched. (The parchment paper will help keep the cake from sticking.)

4. While the cake is baking, spread 3 tablespoons of the confectioners' sugar on a clean kitchen towel. Remove the cake from the oven and invert onto the towel. Peel off the parchment paper and, starting at the short end, roll the cake and towel together. Place on a rack to cool completely.

5. To make the filling, in a blender, combine the ricotta cheese, ¼ cup confectioners' sugar, vanilla extract, and lemon juice, and process until smooth.

6. Gently unroll the cooled cake and spread the filling over the cake to within ½ inch of the edge. Roll the cake up and transfer to a large platter.

7. Cover and refrigerate overnight, or for at least 10 hours. Sift the remaining 2 tablespoons of confectioners' sugar over the roll. Slice and serve.

| | | |
|---|---|---|
| YIELD: 18 SERVINGS | 3.5 G FAT | 40 MG CHOLESTEROL |
| SERVING SIZE: 1 SLICE | 1 G FIBER | 4 G CARBOHYDRATES |
| CALORIES: 112 | 4 G PROTEIN | |
| EXCHANGES: 1 FAT; | | |
| 1 STARCH/BREAD | | |

# Key Lime Cake

❧

*A dense cake, like a pound cake, with a great taste!*

非-stick vegetable cooking spray

1/2 cup sugar

Acesulfame K sugar substitute
equivalent to 1/2 cup sugar

2 cups all-purpose flour

1/2 teaspoon salt

1 teaspoon baking powder

1/2 teaspoon baking soda

1 0.3-ounce package sugar-free lime gelatin

1 1/4 cups canola oil

5 eggs

3/4 cup orange juice, no sugar added

1/4 cup water

1/2 teaspoon vanilla extract

1 teaspoon lemon extract

1/3 cup key lime juice

1/3 cup confectioners' sugar

non-fat whipped topping and
lime slices, for garnish (optional)

1. Preheat oven to 350°. Coat a 9-by-13 inch pan with cooking
   spray.
2. In a large bowl, combine the sugar, sugar substitute, flour,
   salt, baking powder, baking soda, and gelatin. Stir well. Add

the oil, eggs, orange juice, water, and vanilla and lemon extracts. Beat until well blended. Pour into baking pan.

3. Bake 35 to 40 minutes, or until a tester inserted in the center comes out clean. Keep in pan until almost cool, about 15 minutes. Prick cake all over with a fork.

4. In a small bowl, mix together the key lime juice and confectioners' sugar. Drizzle thoroughly over the cooled cake.

5. Cover and refrigerate for 4 to 5 hours, or overnight. Before serving, top with whipped topping and garnish with lime slices, if desired.

YIELD: 20 PIECES          2.9 G FAT               72 MG POTASSIUM
SERVING SIZE: 2 INCHES    0.5 G PROTEIN           50 MG CHOLESTEROL
   BY ½ INCH              4.3 G CARBOHYDRATES
CALORIES: 123

# Lemon-Filled Angel Food Cake

❧

*An ideal party cake that will wow your guests with
its great taste and appearance. Use a purchased cake
or make one from a package or your favorite recipe.*

1 12-inch prepared angel food cake

21 ounces canned lemon pie filling

1 cup low-fat lemon yogurt

1 cup non-fat whipped topping

1. Using a serrated knife, slice the cake horizontally into three layers. In a medium bowl, combine the pie filling and yogurt. Mix well.
2. Frost the first layer with one-third of the lemon mixture. Add the second layer. Frost with half of the remaining lemon mixture. Add the third cake layer. Frost the top of the cake with the remaining lemon mixture.
3. Refrigerate for 2 to 3 hours. Before serving, spread whipped topping over cake.

YIELD: 12 SERVINGS    4 G FAT            40 MG SODIUM
SERVING SIZE: ¹/₁₂ CAKE   1 G FIBER         1 MG CHOLESTEROL
CALORIES: 175       25 G CARBOHYDRATES

# Orange Cake

*A dense yet moist cake.*

1/3 cup sugar

Acesulfame K sugar substitute
equivalent to 1/3 cup sugar

1/2 cup vegetable oil

1 cup sour milk

2 eggs

1 teaspoon baking soda

1 cup unsweetened orange juice
concentrate, thawed

1/4 cup cold water

1/4 teaspoon grated orange peel

2 cups all-purpose flour

1/2 cup chopped walnuts

1/2 cup raisins (optional)

1. Preheat oven to 350°.
2. In a large bowl using an electric mixer, combine the sugar, sugar substitute, oil, sour milk, and eggs. Blend well. Add the baking soda, juice concentrate, water, and orange peel, and blend well. Add the flour and blend until thoroughly combined. Stir in the walnuts and the raisins, if using. Pour into a 9-by-13-inch pan.
3. Bake for 40 to 45 minutes, or until a tester inserted in the center comes out clean.

YIELD: 24 PIECES  8.8 G FAT  14 MG SODIUM
SERVING SIZE: 2¼ INCHES 1 G PROTEIN  60 MG POTASSIUM
  BY 2 INCHES  2.8 G CARBOHYDRATES 0.6 MG CHOLESTEROL
CALORIES: 115

# Pumpkin Cheesecake

*Even if pumpkin is not your
favorite fruit, you will like this.*

1¼ cups all-purpose flour

⅛ cup brown sugar

brown sugar substitute
equivalent to ¼ cup brown sugar

5 tablespoons low-fat margarine

½ cup chopped pecans or walnuts

8 ounces non-fat cream cheese

¼ cup granulated sugar

Acesulfame K sugar substitute
equivalent to ¼ cup sugar

1 cup canned solid-pack pumpkin

1½ teaspoons cinnamon

1 teaspoon nutmeg

½ teaspoon ground cloves

1 teaspoon vanilla extract

1. Preheat oven to 350°.
2. In a medium bowl, combine the flour, brown sugar, and brown sugar substitute. Cut in the margarine. Blend in the nuts. Reserve 1 cup of this mixture. Press remaining mixture into an 8½-by-11-inch pan. Bake for 15 minutes; let it cool slightly.
3. While the crust is baking, in a medium bowl using an electric mixer, blend the cream cheese, granulated sugar, sugar

substitute, pumpkin, cinnamon, nutmeg, cloves, and vanilla extract until smooth. Stir well and pour over the crust. Sprinkle with the reserved topping.

4. Bake for 30 to 35 minutes, or until a tester inserted in the center comes out clean.

YIELD: 24 PIECES
SERVING SIZE: 2 INCHES
   BY 1¾ INCHES
CALORIES: 75

3.5 G FAT
1.5 G PROTEIN
2 G CARBOHYDRATES

10 MG SODIUM
11 MG CHOLESTEROL

# Apple Cake

⁂

*This cake has a dense, spongy texture.*

non-stick vegetable cooking spray

3 egg whites

2 cups all-purpose flour

1/2 cup sugar

Acesulfame K sugar substitute equivalent to 1/3 cup sugar

1/2 teaspoon baking soda

1 teaspoon cinnamon

1/2 cup nutmeg

1 cup unsweetened applesauce

1 teaspoon vanilla extract

2 large apples, peeled and chopped

1. Preheat oven to 350°. Coat a 9-by-13-inch pan with non-stick cooking spray.
2. In a small bowl using an electric mixer, beat the egg whites until stiff peaks form. In a large bowl, mix the flour, sugar, sugar substitute, baking soda, cinnamon, and nutmeg. Add the applesauce and vanilla extract to dry mixture and blend well. Fold in the egg whites and mix thoroughly. Stir in the apples and blend well. Pour into the prepared pan.
3. Bake for 35 to 40 minutes, or until a tester inserted in the center comes out clean.

YIELD: 15 SERVINGS          TRACE FAT
SERVING SIZE: 2 INCHES BY 4 INCHES
CALORIES: 120

# Fruit-Topped Low-Fat Lemon Cheesecake

*Use your favorite fresh seasonal fruit such as raspberries, strawberries, peaches, blueberries, or whatever you like to top this creation.*

non-stick vegetable cooking spray

¼ cup graham cracker crumbs

8 ounces non-fat cream cheese

1 14-ounce can non-fat sweetened condensed milk

3 egg whites

1 whole egg

⅓ cup lemon juice concentrate, thawed

1 teaspoon vanilla extract

¼ cup all-purpose flour

1 cup seasonal fresh fruit

1. Preheat oven to 300°. Coat the bottom of an angel food cake pan with non-stick cooking spray.
2. Sprinkle the graham cracker crumbs evenly on bottom of pan. In a large bowl using an electric mixer, beat the cream cheese until fluffy. Gradually add the condensed milk and beat until smooth. Add the egg whites, whole egg, juice concentrate, and vanilla extract. Stir in the flour. Blend well. Pour into the prepared pan.
3. Bake for 45 to 50 minutes, or until a tester inserted in center comes out clean. Cool. Refrigerate for 3 to 4 hours. Top with fresh fruit before serving.

YIELD: 10 SERVINGS     2 G FAT              375 MG SODIUM
SERVING SIZE: ¹⁄₁₀ CAKE   12 G PROTEIN         30 MG CHOLESTEROL
CALORIES: 200          30 G CARBOHYDRATES

# Chocolate Cheesecake

*Note: May be served topped with whipped topping or with strawberries. If these are used, be sure to add the calories to servings.*

non-stick vegetable cooking spray

2 cups non-fat cottage cheese

2 eggs

⅓ cup sugar

Acesulfame K sugar substitute equivalent to ⅓ cup sugar

4 ounces Neufchâtel cheese, softened

⅓ cup cocoa

1 teaspoon vanilla extract

1. Preheat oven to 300°. Coat an 8¼-by-12¼-inch cake pan or a 9-inch springform pan with non-stick cooking spray.
2. In a large bowl using an electric mixer, blend the cottage cheese, eggs, sugar, sugar substitute, Neufchâtel cheese, cocoa, and vanilla extract until smooth. Pour into the prepared pan.
3. Bake for 35 minutes, or until edges are set. Cool completely on a wire rack.
4. Refrigerate for 4 hours, or until chilled.

YIELD: 12 PIECES
SERVING SIZE: 2¾ INCHES BY 3 INCHES
CALORIES: 130

3 G FAT
8 G PROTEIN
17 G CARBOHYDRATES

240 MG SODIUM
8 MG CHOLESTEROL

# Lemon Delight

*This soufflé-style dessert is an old recipe from my
mother and her friend, Mrs. E. Johnson. It had a lot
of sugar in it. I modified it so that it fits into a diabetic
diet and is still a great tasting, refreshing dessert.*

> 2 tablespoons low-fat margarine
>
> ¼ cup sugar
>
> Acesulfame K sugar substitute
> equivalent to ¼ cup sugar
>
> 2 egg yolks
>
> 2 tablespoons all-purpose flour
>
> 3 tablespoons lemon juice
>
> 1 cup 2% milk
>
> 2 egg whites, chilled

1. Preheat oven to 350°.
2. In a medium bowl, cream the margarine, sugar, and sugar substitute until well blended. Add the egg yolks and beat well. Blend in the flour. Add the lemon juice, then slowly add the milk, stirring constantly.
3. In a small bowl using an electric mixer, beat the egg whites until stiff peaks form. Fold the egg whites into the margarine mixture and gently mix until well blended. Pour into a soufflé dish and place in a larger pan of hot water.
4. Bake for 40 to 45 minutes, or until lightly browned. Cool slightly. Serve at once, or refrigerate and serve chilled.

| | | |
|---|---|---|
| YIELD: 6 SERVINGS | 3 G FAT | 34.2 MG SODIUM |
| SERVING SIZE: ⅙ SOUFFLÉ | 3.5 G PROTEIN | 75 MG CHOLESTEROL |
| CALORIES: 60 | 6.5 G CARBOHYDRATES | |

# PIES

## Tips for Baking Pies

- When baking fruit pies, if the juice runs over, shake salt on the spills. They will burn to a crisp and will be easily cleaned away with a spatula.
- To keep apples from discoloring, sprinkle with lemon juice or put them in water with a little lemon juice. Drain before using them.
- For bananas, sprinkle lightly with lemon juice.
- Unbaked frozen pie shells can go from the freezer straight to the oven without thawing.
- To heat baked frozen fruit pies, let stand for 30 minutes and then place in a 350° oven for 10 minutes to warm. Place a pan or aluminum foil under the pan to catch the spills. A piece of pie may be warmed for a few seconds in the microwave.
- Unflavored gelatin comes in a box of envelopes. Each envelope contains 1 tablespoon of gelatin.

# Custard Pie

3 eggs, lightly beaten

2 tablespoons sugar

¼ teaspoon salt

½ teaspoon nutmeg

2 cups non-fat milk

1 teaspoon vanilla extract

1 8-inch prepared pie crust, unbaked

¼ teaspoon cinnamon

1. Preheat oven to 325°.
2. In a medium bowl, combine the eggs, sugar, salt, and nutmeg. Slowly stir in the milk and vanilla extract. Pour into the prepared pie shell. Sprinkle with the cinnamon.
3. Bake for 45 minutes, or until a tester inserted in the center comes out clean.

YIELD: 6 SERVINGS
SERVING SIZE: ⅙ PIE
CALORIES: 183

7.5 G FAT
6.8 G PROTEIN
23 G CARBOHYDRATES

205.3 MG SODIUM
167.8 MG POTASSIUM
138 MG CHOLESTEROL

# Apple Crisp

non-stick vegetable cooking spray

3 large Ida Red or Cortland apples,
peeled and sliced

¼ cup rolled oats

1 tablespoon all-purpose flour

1 tablespoon low-fat margarine,
cut into small pieces

1 tablespoon sugar

1 teaspoon cinnamon

1. Preheat oven to 350°. Coat an 8-inch square pan with non-stick cooking spray.
2. Place the apple slices in the prepared pan. In a medium bowl, combine the oats, flour, margarine, sugar, and cinnamon. Stir until crumbly. Sprinkle over the apple slices.
3. Bake for 25 minutes, or until golden brown.

YIELD: 4 SERVINGS     4 G FAT     179 MG SODIUM
SERVING SIZE: 4 INCHES     2 G PROTEIN     31 G CARBOHYDRATES
    BY 4 INCHES
CALORIES: 230
EXCHANGES: 1 FAT; 2 FRUIT;
    1 STARCH/BREAD

# Crunchy Apple Cobbler

❧

*Crunchy and delicious,*
*a cobbler I like served warm.*

non-stick vegetable cooking spray

$\frac{1}{2}$ cup rolled oats

6 cups thinly sliced Ida Red or Cortland apples

$\frac{1}{2}$ cup frozen unsweetened apple juice concentrate, thawed

$\frac{1}{4}$ teaspoon cloves, ground

1 teaspoon cinnamon

2 tablespoons raisins (optional)

$\frac{1}{3}$ cup bran flakes cereal

1. Preheat oven to 350°. Coat an 8-inch square pan with non-stick cooking spray.
2. Layer the oats in the bottom of the pan. Add the apple slices. In a measuring cup, combine the juice concentrate, cloves, and cinnamon. Pour over the apples and oats. Sprinkle raisins on top, if desired. Cover with foil.
3. Bake for 1 hour. Remove foil. Sprinkle the top of mixture with the cereal and bake for 10 minutes longer. Serve hot or cold.

YIELD: 6 SERVINGS
SERVING SIZE: $2\frac{2}{3}$ INCHES BY $2\frac{2}{3}$ INCHES
CALORIES: 150
EXCHANGES: 2 FRUIT; $\frac{1}{2}$ STARCH/BREAD

# Peach Betty

*You can make this dessert a day ahead
and serve it hot or cold.*

29 ounces canned all natural
   sliced peaches
½ teaspoon cinnamon
¼ teaspoon nutmeg
 1 teaspoon grated lemon peel
 1 tablespoon low-fat margarine
⅓ cup finely crushed cornflakes

1. Preheat oven to 375°.
2. In an 8-inch baking dish, combine the peaches, cinnamon, nutmeg, and lemon peel. In a small saucepan over low heat, melt the margarine. Add the cornflakes and mix well. Sprinkle the crumb mixture over the peaches.
3. Bake for 30 to 35 minutes, or until heated through and the crumbs are brown.

YIELD: 4 SERVINGS
SERVING SIZE: 4 INCHES BY 4 INCHES
CALORIES: 105 PER SERVING
EXCHANGES: ¼ FAT; 1 FRUIT; ½ STARCH/BREAD

# Baked Rhubarb Strawberry Pie

*To keep filling from leaking through a baked pie crust,
brush the crust with a lightly beaten egg yolk to
seal prick holes. Microwave for 30 to 40 seconds to set.*

¼ cup sugar

Acesulfame K sugar substitute
equivalent to ¼ cup sugar

¼ cup all-purpose flour

2 cups rhubarb, cut into small pieces

1 8-inch prepared pie crust, unbaked

1½ cups sliced strawberries

1. Preheat oven to 350°.
2. In a small bowl, mix together the sugar, sugar substitute, and flour. Place a thin layer of the rhubarb in the unbaked pie crust. Sprinkle 2 tablespoons of the sugar mixture over this layer. In a medium bowl, combine the remaining rhubarb and the strawberries. Gently fold in the remaining sugar mixture. Blend well. Spoon on top of the mixture in the crust. Cover with aluminum foil.
3. Bake for 35 minutes. Remove foil and bake uncovered for 20 to 25 minutes longer, or until pie shell edges are golden brown. Cool before serving.

YIELD: 8 SERVINGS     1 G FAT     8 MG SODIUM
SERVING SIZE: ⅛ PIE     1 G FIBER
CALORIES: 60     3 G CARBOHYDRATES

# No Bake Strawberry Rhubarb Pie

2 cups rhubarb, cut into small pieces

⅛ cup sugar

Acesulfame K sugar substitute
equivalent to ¼ cup sugar

¼ cup water

1¼ cups sliced strawberries

3 packets Acesulfame K sugar substitute

1 0.3-ounce package sugar-free
strawberry gelatin

1 8-inch shortbread crust

1. In a saucepan over medium heat, combine rhubarb, sugar, the ¼ cup equivalent of sugar substitute, and the water.
2. Cook for 15 minutes, or until the rhubarb is soft. Stir in the strawberries, remaining sugar substitute, and gelatin. Pour into the prepared crust.
3. Refrigerate for 4 to 5 hours, or until firm.

YIELD: 8 SERVINGS     3 G FAT     6 G CARBOHYDRATES
SERVING SIZE: ⅛ PIE     1 G FIBER     1 G PROTEIN
CALORIES: 60

# Peach Pie

3 tablespoons tapioca

6 ounces unsweetened white grape juice

2 tablespoons lemon juice

⅛ teaspoon salt

4 cups thinly sliced fresh peaches

1 8-inch prepared pie crust

3 tablespoons all-purpose flour

1 packet Acesulfame K sugar substitute

2 tablespoons low-fat margarine

1. Preheat oven to 400°.
2. In a medium saucepan, mix the tapioca into the white grape juice and let soak for 10 minutes. Add the lemon juice and salt and cook over medium heat, stirring constantly, until thickened.
3. Place the peaches in a large bowl and pour in the tapioca mixture. Blend well. Pour into the prepared pie shell.
4. In a small bowl, mix together the flour, sugar substitute, and margarine. Spoon the topping on the peaches. Cover with foil.
5. Bake for 10 minutes. Reduce heat to 350° and bake for 40 to 45 minutes longer, removing foil for the last 10 minutes.

YIELD: 8 SERVINGS
SERVING SIZE: ⅛ PIE
CALORIES: 240
EXCHANGES: 2 FAT; 1½ FRUIT;
   1 STARCH/BREAD

12 G FAT
3 G PROTEIN
25 G CARBOHYDRATES

# Apple Surprise

*Appealing in taste, texture, and appearance,*
*this fabulous dessert was a favorite at our R&D events.*

  1 tablespoon low-fat margarine
  1 package white cake mix with
    pudding in mix
  ½ cup low-fat margarine, melted
  1¼ cups rolled quick oats
  1 egg
  6 apples, peeled and sliced
  ½ cup chopped pecans
    brown sugar substitute equivalent
    to ¼ cup brown sugar

1. Preheat oven to 350°. Grease a 9-by-13-inch cake pan.
2. In a large bowl, combine the cake mix, 6 tablespoons of the melted margarine, and 1 cup of the oats. Mix until crumbly. Reserve 1 cup for topping.
3. To remaining crumbs, add the egg. Mix until well blended. Press into the prepared pan. Place sliced apples evenly over crust.
4. To the reserved crumbs, add the remaining oats, remaining margarine, nuts, and brown sugar substitute. Blend until thoroughly mixed. Sprinkle over apple mixture.
4. Bake for 45 to 50 minutes. Serve warm or cold.

YIELD: 15 SERVINGS    10 G FAT        22 MG SODIUM
SERVING SIZE: 3 INCHES    0.6 G PROTEIN    5.6 G CARBOHYDRATES
  BY 2½ INCHES    0.4 G FIBER
CALORIES: 184

# Lime Pie

❧

*About 14 graham crackers (rectangles)*
*makes 1⅔ cups crushed graham crackers.*

1⅔ cups graham cracker crumbs

¼ cup low-fat margarine, melted

⅛ cup sugar

Acesulfame K sugar substitute
equivalent to ⅛ cup sugar

1 envelope (1 tablespoon) Knox™
unflavored gelatin

½ cup cold water

8 ounces low-fat lime yogurt

½ cup non-fat mayonnaise

1 cup non-fat whipped topping, thawed

1. Preheat oven to 350°.
2. In a medium bowl, mix together the graham cracker crumbs, margarine, sugar, and sugar substitute. Press into the bottom and up the sides of a 9-inch pie pan. Bake for 8 to 10 minutes. Remove from oven and cool.
3. In a saucepan, combine the gelatin and water. Heat on low, stirring until dissolved. Remove from heat. Add the yogurt and mayonnaise and beat, using an electric mixer at medium speed, until well blended. Fold in the whipped topping. Pour into the prepared crust.
4. Refrigerate for 2 hours, or until firm.

YIELD: 8 SERVINGS          5 G FAT          5 MG CHOLESTEROL
SERVING SIZE: ⅛ PIE
CALORIES: 170

# Lemon Pie

*A shortbread crust is very good for this pie.*

¼ cup sugar

6 packets Acesulfame K sugar substitute

1 tablespoon cornstarch

⅓ cup lemon juice

⅓ cup cold water

1 large egg yolk

1 teaspoon grated lemon peel

1 envelope (1 tablespoon) Knox™ unflavored gelatin

1¼ cups 2% milk

1 teaspoon vanilla extract

⅓ cup non-fat whipped topping, thawed

1 8-inch prepared pie crust

1. Boil water in the bottom of a double boiler.
2. In the top of a double boiler, combine the sugar, sugar substitute, and cornstarch. Whisk in the lemon juice, water, egg yolk, and lemon peel until well blended. Cook over boiling water, stirring constantly, for 5 minutes. Refrigerate for 30 minutes, or until well chilled.
3. In a saucepan, sprinkle the gelatin over ¼ cup of the milk to soften it. Cook over low heat until the gelatin dissolves. Pour into a large bowl. Add the remaining milk and vanilla extract. Refrigerate until the mixture begins to gel.

4. Using an electric mixer, beat the chilled sugar mixture until fluffy. Fold in the whipped topping, then fold this mixture into the gelatin mixture. Blend well. Spoon into the prepared crust.

5. Chill for 1 hour.

YIELD: 8 SERVINGS
SERVING SIZE: ⅛ PIE
CALORIES: 120
EXCHANGES: 3 FAT; 1 FRUIT; 1 STARCH/BREAD

# Pumpkin Chiffon Pie

1 ounce instant sugar-free vanilla pudding

½ teaspoon cinnamon

¼ teaspoon ground ginger

½ teaspoon nutmeg

15 ounces canned solid-pack pumpkin

½ cup 2% milk

⅛ cup water

2 egg whites

⅛ cup sugar

2 packets Acesulfame K sugar substitute

1 8-inch prepared graham cracker or shortbread pie crust

½ cup non-fat whipped topping

1. In a large bowl using an electric mixer on low speed, blend the pudding mix, spices, pumpkin, milk, and water for 3 to 4 minutes until well combined. In a medium bowl, beat the egg whites until frothy. Gradually add the sugar and sugar substitute, beating constantly, until soft peaks form. Fold in the pudding mixture. Pour into the prepared crust.

2. Refrigerate for 4 hours. Top each serving with 1 tablespoon of the whipped topping.

YIELD: 8 SERVINGS      2 G FAT
SERVING SIZE: ⅛ PIE      1 G FIBER
CALORIES: 75      1 G CARBOHYDRATES

# Baked Pumpkin Pie

⅓ cup sugar

Acesulfame K sugar substitute equivalent to ⅓ cup sugar

15 ounces canned solid-pack pumpkin

1 teaspoon vanilla extract

1½ cups evaporated non-fat milk

2 eggs, beaten

1 teaspoon cinnamon

½ teaspoon ground ginger

½ teaspoon nutmeg

¼ teaspoon cloves, ground

1 8-inch prepared graham cracker crust

1. Preheat oven to 400°.
2. In a large bowl, combine the sugar, sugar substitute, pumpkin, and vanilla extract. Mix until smooth. Add the milk and eggs and mix again. Stir in the cinnamon, ginger, nutmeg, and cloves. Mix well. Pour into the prepared pie shell.
3. Bake at 400° for 10 minutes. Reduce heat to 325° and bake for 45 minutes longer, or until a tester inserted in the center comes out clean.

YIELD: 8 SERVINGS    5 G FAT
SERVING SIZE: ⅛ PIE    1 G CARBOHYDRATES
CALORIES: 125

# Cherry Pineapple Fluff

21 ounces canned lite cherry pie filling

12 ounces canned non-fat sweetened condensed milk

20 ounces canned crushed pineapple (in its own juice)

2 cups non-fat whipped topping

1. In a large bowl, combine the pie filling and milk. Mix well. Add the pineapple and mix again. Fold in the whipped topping. Spoon into 8 sherbet glasses.
2. Refrigerate overnight.

YIELD: 8 SERVINGS     1 G FAT     22 MG SODIUM
SERVING SIZE: 1 CUP     0.5 G PROTEIN     18 G CARBOHYDRATES
CALORIES: 150

# Coconut Pineapple Dream Pie

non-stick vegetable cooking spray

1 cup flaked coconut

15¼ ounces canned crushed
pineapple (in its own juice)

1 cup egg substitute

6 packets Acesulfame K sugar substitute

1 cup 2% milk

½ cup low-fat baking mix

1 teaspoon vanilla extract

1. Preheat oven to 350°. Coat a 9-inch pie pan with non-stick cooking spray.
2. Sprinkle the coconut over bottom of the prepared pan. Drain the pineapple reserving the juice. Place the pineapple over the coconut and set aside.
3. In a blender, blend the egg substitute and sugar substitute. Add the milk, reserved pineapple juice, baking mix, and vanilla extract and process at medium speed until well blended. Pour mixture over pineapple in pie pan.
4. Bake for 35 minutes, or until a tester inserted in the center comes out clean.
5. Refrigerate until serving.

YIELD: 8 SERVINGS    8 G FAT    165 MG SODIUM
SERVING SIZE: ⅛ PIE    5 G PROTEIN    2 MG CHOLESTEROL
CALORIES: 163    18 G CARBOHYDRATES

# Fresh Raspberry Pie

1 1/2 cups water

1 tablespoon cornstarch

4 packets Acesulfame K
sugar substitute

1 0.3-ounce package sugar-free
raspberry gelatin

4 cups fresh raspberries

1 9-inch prepared pie crust,
pre-baked

1. In a medium saucepan over medium heat, mix the water and cornstarch. Cook, stirring constantly, until bubbles form.
2. Remove from heat. Sprinkle the sugar substitute and gelatin over the mixture.
3. Stir and let cool. Fold in the raspberries. Pour into the prepared crust.

YIELD: 8 SERVINGS
SERVING SIZE: 1/8 PIE
CALORIES: 115
EXCHANGES: 1 FAT; 1 FRUIT; 1 STARCH/BREAD

# Strawberry Chiffon Pie

   1 1-ounce package sugar-free,
      fat-free vanilla pudding mix (instant)

1 ¼ cups 2% milk

   8 ounces non-fat lemon chiffon yogurt

   4 cups fresh sliced strawberries

   1 8-inch prepared shortbread crust


1. Prepare pudding mix with milk; blend for 2 minutes with an electric mixer on medium speed.
2. Add yogurt and mix well with a spoon. Fold in 3 cups of the strawberries. Pour into the prepared crust.
3. Top with remaining strawberries.

YIELD: 8 SERVINGS     2 G FAT         130 MG SODIUM
SERVING SIZE: ⅛ PIE    2 G PROTEIN    TRACE CHOLESTEROL
CALORIES: 135        6.5 G CARBOHYDRATES

# Rhubarb Dessert

½ cup low-fat margarine

2 cups all-purpose flour

2½ teaspoons baking powder

¼ teaspoon salt

⅛ cup brown sugar

brown sugar substitute equivalent to ⅛ cup brown sugar

1 egg, beaten

¾ cup 2% milk

4 cups finely chopped rhubarb

6 tablespoons low-fat margarine

½ cup granulated sugar

Acesulfame K sugar substitute equivalent to ½ cup sugar

2 tablespoons all-purpose flour

1 0.3-ounce package sugar-free strawberry gelatin

1. Preheat oven to 350°.
2. In a medium bowl, mix together the margarine, flour, baking powder, and salt. Add the brown sugar and brown sugar substitute. Add the egg and milk and mix well. Spread into the bottom and up the sides of a 9-by-13-inch pan.
3. Place the rhubarb in a large bowl. In a small bowl, mix together the margarine, granulated sugar, sugar substitute, and flour. Mix until crumbly. Sprinkle the margarine mix-

ture and gelatin on top of the rhubarb. Pour the rhubarb mixture over the mixture in the pan.

4. Bake for 45 to 50 minutes, or until a tester inserted in the center comes out clean.

YIELD: 24 SERVINGS
SERVING SIZE: 2¼ INCHES BY 2¼ INCHES
CALORIES: 90

3 G FAT
1 G PROTEIN
5 G CARBOHYDRATES

# Cherry Special Dessert

*Fantastic! A favorite dessert with a great taste.*

1 tablespoon low-fat margarine

1 package white cake mix with pudding in mix

1/2 cup low-fat margarine, melted

1 1/4 cups rolled quick oats

1 egg

20 ounces canned lite cherry pie filling

1/2 cup chopped walnuts

brown sugar substitute
equivalent to 1/4 cup brown sugar

1. Preheat oven to 350°. Grease a 9-by-13-inch pan.
2. In a large bowl, combine the cake mix, 6 tablespoons of the margarine, and 1 cup of the oats. Mix until crumbly. Reserve 1 cup crumbs for topping. To the remaining crumbs, add the egg and mix until well blended. Press into prepared pan. Pour pie filling over crust and spread evenly.
3. To the reserved crumbs, add the remaining oats and margarine, nuts, and brown sugar substitute. Blend until thoroughly mixed. Sprinkle over the cherry mixture.
4. Bake for 45 to 50 minutes. Serve warm or cold.

YIELD: 15 SERVINGS    10 G FAT    12 MG SODIUM
SERVING SIZE: 3 INCHES    0.4 G FIBER    0.6 G PROTEIN
   BY 2 1/2 INCHES    5.6 G CARBOHYDRATES
CALORIES: 181
NOTE: CONTAINS 2 G SUGAR

# No-Bake Sugar-Free Pumpkin Pie

✿

1 9-inch pie crust

1 envelope (1 tablespoon) Knox™ unflavored gelatin

1/3 cup cold water

2 cups 2% milk

1 ounce instant sugar-free butterscotch pudding

1 tablespoon pumpkin pie spice

1 teaspoon cinnamon

1/2 teaspoon nutmeg

2 packets Acesulfame K sugar substitute

16 ounces canned solid-pack pumpkin

1. Bake the pie crust according to package directions. Cool.
2. In a measuring cup, soften the gelatin in the cold water until mushy. Set in pan of hot water until transparent.
3. In a large bowl using an electric mixer, beat the milk and the pudding mix until smooth. Add the gelatin mixture, spices, and sugar substitute beating constantly until smooth. Add the pumpkin and beat for 2 minutes longer or until thoroughly mixed. Pour into prepared pie crust.
4. Refrigerate for at least 8 hours or overnight.

YIELD: 6 SERVINGS     3 G FAT     60 MG SODIUM
SERVING SIZE: 1/6 PIE     1 G FIBER     2 MG CHOLESTEROL
CALORIES: 108

# Fruit Concoctions

## Fruit Quantities

**Apples:** 1 pound = 2 large, 3 medium, 4 small; 2¾ cups sliced; 3 cups diced

**Bananas:** 1 pound = 2 large, 3 medium; ⅓ cup mashed; 1½ cups diced

**Grapes:** 60 Thompson seedless = ½ cup

**Lemons:** 1 medium = 3 teaspoons grated peel; 3 tablespoons juice

**Limes:** 1 medium = 2 teaspoons grated peel; 2 tablespoons juice

**Oranges:** 1 medium = 10 to 11 sections; 4 teaspoons grated peel; ⅓ cup juice

**Peaches:** 1 pound = 2 large; 3 medium; 2 cups sliced; 1⅔ cups diced

**Pears:** 1 pound = 2 large, 3 medium; 2½ cups sliced; 2⅓ cups diced

**Plums:** 1 pound = 6 medium; 2½ cups sliced; 2 cups diced

**Strawberries:** 1 quart = about 6½ cups whole; about 4½ cups sliced

**Tangerines:** 1 medium = 3 to 4 teaspoons juice; 2 to 3 teaspoons grated peel

# Apple Pineapple Salad

6 ounces unsweetened frozen
  orange juice concentrate, thawed

1 cup cold water

4 apples, peeled and chopped

16 ounces canned crushed
  pineapple (in its own juice)

1 packet Acesulfame K (or
  2 teaspoons other sugar substitute)

1. In a large bowl, combine the orange juice concentrate and water. Add the apples, pineapple, and sugar substitute. Blend well.
2. Refrigerate for 30 minutes before serving.

YIELD: 10 SERVINGS      1 G PROTEIN               2 MG SODIUM
SERVING SIZE: ½ CUP     20 G CARBOHYDRATES
CALORIES: 83
EXCHANGES: 1½ FRUIT

# Melon Ball Salad

¹/₃ cup each honeydew, cantaloupe,
and watermelon balls

1. Cut a honeydew and a cantaloupe in half. Clean out the seeds. Then ball part of one-half of each melon. Slice off a 2-inch slice of watermelon. Take out seeds. Then ball part of this slice.
2. Refrigerate for 30 minutes before serving.

YIELD: 1 SERVING        15 G CARBOHYDRATES
SERVING SIZE: 1 CUP
CALORIES: 60
EXCHANGES: 1 FRUIT

# Lime Applesauce Mold

❧

*When you unmold gelatin, wet the dish on*
*which the gelatin is to be unmolded,*
*and it can be moved around until centered.*

15 ounces unsweetened applesauce

1 0.3-ounce package sugar-free lime gelatin

8 ounces canned crushed pineapple
(in its own juice)

7 ounces sugar-free lemon-lime soda

1. In saucepan, combine the applesauce and gelatin. Cook, stirring until the gelatin dissolves. Cool to room temperature.
2. Add the pineapple and stir well. Gently stir in soda. Pour into gelatin mold.
3. Refrigerate for 4 hours, or until set. Unmold to serve.

YIELD: 4 SERVINGS     TRACE PROTEIN     55 MG SODIUM
SERVING SIZE: ½ CUP     12 G CARBOHYDRATES
CALORIES: 120

# Molded Melon Salad

*Ginger adds a mild spice to this
deliciously different combination.*

1 cup boiling water

1 0.3-ounce package sugar-free
orange gelatin

³/₄ cup frozen unsweetened
orange juice concentrate, thawed

¹/₈ teaspoon powdered ginger

1 cup honeydew balls or small chunks

1 cup cantaloupe or watermelon
balls or small chunks

1. In a large bowl, pour the boiling water over the gelatin and stir until dissolved. Stir in the orange juice concentrate and ginger. Refrigerate for 45 minutes, or until slightly thickened.
2. Stir in the melon. Pour into gelatin mold.
3. Refrigerate for 4 to 5 hours, or until set. Unmold to serve.

YIELD: 6 SERVINGS       6 G CARBOHYDRATES
SERVING SIZE: ³/₄ CUP
CALORIES: 56
EXCHANGE: 1 FRUIT

# Lemon Gelatin Salad with Pears and Pineapple

    1 1/2  cups boiling water
       2  0.3-ounce packages
           sugar-free lemon gelatin
    1 1/2  cups cold water
       8  ounces low-fat key lime yogurt
   15 1/2  ounces canned sliced lite
           pears drained (in its own juice)
   15 1/2  ounces canned crushed pineapple
           (in its own juice)
       1  4-ounce jar green maraschino
           cherries, drained

1. In a large bowl, pour the boiling water over the lemon gelatin and stir until gelatin is dissolved. Stir in the cold water. Pour half the gelatin mixture into a 9-by-13-inch pan. Refrigerate for 45 minutes, or until thickened.
2. Spread the yogurt over the thickened mixture. Layer pear slices on top of yogurt. To the remaining gelatin, stir in the pineapple and cherries. Pour the pineapple mixture over the pears.
3. Refrigerate for 3 to 4 hours, or until firm.

YIELD: 12 SERVINGS          1 G FAT              95 MG SODIUM
SERVING SIZE: 3 INCHES      6 G PROTEIN          200 MG POTASSIUM
    BY 4 INCHES             7 G CARBOHYDRATES    5 MG CHOLESTEROL
CALORIES: 88

# Lime Yogurt Gelatin Salad

*Pears and lime are a surprisingly tasty combination.
The cool citrus was very well liked at our R&D luncheons.*

15 ounces canned lite pears
(reserve juice)

2 cups boiling water

2 0.3-ounce packages
sugar-free lime gelatin

8 ounces non-fat vanilla yogurt

1. Drain the pears, reserving ½ cup juice. Slice pears. In a small bowl, pour the boiling water over the gelatin and stir until gelatin is dissolved. Measure 1 cup of gelatin mixture and blend with the yogurt. Pour into an 8-inch square pan. Chill until thickened but not firm.
2. To the remaining gelatin, add the reserved pear juice and chill until slightly thickened. Arrange the pear slices on the gelatin and yogurt mixture. Top with the clear gelatin mixture.
3. Refrigerate for 3 to 4 hours, or until firm.

YIELD: 8 SERVINGS
SERVING SIZE: 2 INCHES
  BY 4 INCHES
CALORIES: 60

0.6 G PROTEIN
8.5 G CARBOHYDRATES

11 MG SODIUM
31 MG POTASSIUM

# Molded Waldorf Salad

*Here you'll find the flavors of a traditional
Waldorf salad in a gelatin mold. Delicious!*

1 0.3-ounce package sugar-free
   lemon gelatin

1 cup boiling water

8 ounces canned crushed pineapple
   (in its own juice)

8 ounces canned mandarin oranges,
   partially drained

1 banana, sliced

1 apple, chopped

¼ cup grapes

½ cup chopped walnuts or pecans

1. In a large bowl, pour the boiling water over the gelatin and
   stir until the gelatin dissolves. Add the pineapple with juice,
   oranges, banana, apple, grapes, and nuts. Mix well. Pour
   into an 8-inch square pan.
2. Refrigerate for 3 to 4 hours, or until firm.

YIELD: 8 SERVINGS     0.5 G FAT     7 MG SODIUM
SERVING SIZE: 2 INCHES     18 G CARBOHYDRATES     78 MG POTASSIUM
   BY 4 INCHES
CALORIES: 93

# Banana Pineapple Frozen Salad

2 cups low-fat sour cream

¼ cup sugar

Acesulfame K sugar substitute
equivalent to ¼ cup sugar

3 tablespoons lemon juice

8 ounces canned crushed pineapple,
drained (in its own juice)

3 bananas, sliced

8 maraschino cherries cut into halves

1. In a bowl, combine the sour cream, sugar, sugar substitute, lemon juice, pineapple, and banana. Mix very well. Pour into a 9-by-13-inch pan.
2. Freeze for at least 4 hours. Garnish each serving with a cherry half.

YIELD: 15 SERVINGS

SERVING SIZE: 3 INCHES
BY 2½ INCHES

CALORIES: 75

3 G FAT

125 MG POTASSIUM

9 G CARBOHYDRATES

4 MG SODIUM

10 MG CHOLESTEROL

# Sugar-Free Fruit Salad

❧

 1 1-ounce package sugar-free,
   fat-free vanilla instant pudding mix

1½ cups 2% milk

 16 ounces canned mixed fruit,
   drained (in its own juice)

 13 ounces canned pineapple chunks,
   drained (in its own juice)

 11 ounces canned mandarin oranges,
   drained and rinsed

1. In a large bowl, using an electric beater, mix the instant pudding and milk. Add drained fruits and gently stir together.
2. Refrigerate for 2 to 3 hours, or until pudding is set.

YIELD: 6 SERVINGS    1 G FAT     140 MG SODIUM
SERVING SIZE: ½ CUP   1 G FIBER     5 MG CHOLESTEROL
CALORIES: 147     30 G CARBOHYDRATES

# Royal Anne Cherry Salad

*This lovely salad makes a beautiful
addition to your holiday table.*

8 ounces non-fat cream cheese

14 ounces canned Royal Anne cherries,
pitted and drained, reserving juice

¼ cup cold water

1 cup boiling water

1 0.3-ounce package sugar-free cherry gelatin

8 ounces non-fat whipped topping, thawed

1. In a bowl, combine the cream cheese, 2 tablespoons of the reserved cherry juice, and cold water. Beat well using an electric mixer.
2. In a separate bowl, pour the boiling water over the gelatin and stir until the gelatin dissolves. Add to the cream cheese mixture and blend well. Fold in drained cherries and whipped topping. Pour into a 9-by-13-inch pan.
3. Refrigerate for several hours or overnight.

YIELD: 9 SERVINGS
SERVING SIZE: 3 INCHES BY 4 INCHES
CALORIES: 110

2 G FIBER
20 G CARBOHYDRATES

# Frozen Fruit Salad

*A frozen salad is an excellent
choice to make ahead for a party.*

8 ounces cream cheese

2 tablespoons 2% milk

⅓ cup mayonnaise

2 tablespoons lemon juice

15 ounces canned Mandarin orange
sections, drained and sliced

1 cup canned crushed pineapple
(in its own juice)

½ cup Royal Anne cherries,
pitted and chopped

½ cup red maraschino cherries

½ cup pecans

8 ounces non-fat whipped topping, thawed

1. In a bowl, mix the cream cheese with the milk. Stir in the mayonnaise and lemon juice. Add the oranges, pineapple, cherries, and nuts. Fold in the whipped topping. Place in a 9-by-13-inch pan.
2. Freeze for 1 hour, or until firm.

YIELD: 20 SERVINGS
SERVING SIZE: 2 INCHES
   BY 2¾ INCHES
CALORIES: 108

3 G FAT
0.5 G FIBER
2 G PROTEIN

50 MG SODIUM
3 MG CHOLESTEROL
12 G CARBOHYDRATES

# In the Pink Salad

🌿

*Its slightly tart taste makes this
a good side dish with the main meal.*

20 ounces canned crushed pineapple
(in its own juice)

2 0.3-ounce packages sugar-free
strawberry gelatin

1 cup sugar-free cherry juice

1/4 teaspoon nutmeg

3 tablespoons lemon juice

1/2 cup chopped pecans

2 cups low-fat sour cream

1. Drain pineapple well, reserving fruit and juice separately. In
   a small saucepan, add the pineapple juice to the gelatin. Stir
   in the cherry juice and heat to boiling, stirring constantly to
   dissolve gelatin. Remove from heat. Stir in the nutmeg and
   lemon juice. Chill until mixture thickens slightly.

2. Stir in pecans and sour cream. Add the reserved pineapple
   and stir again. Pour into a 9-by-13-inch pan.

3. Refrigerate until firm.

YIELD: 16 SERVINGS     2 G FAT         58 MG SODIUM
SERVING SIZE: 2 INCHES    1 G PROTEIN
    BY 3 INCHES        8 G CARBOHYDRATES
CALORIES: 60

# Lime Sour Cream Salad

  1 cup boiling water
  2 0.3-ounce packages sugar-free
    lime gelatin
  2 cups non-fat sour cream
 20 ounces canned crushed pineapple
    (in its own juice)
  8 ounces non-fat key lime yogurt
 ½ cup maraschino cherries
 ½ cup chopped pecans

1. In a large bowl, pour the boiling water over the gelatin and stir until the gelatin dissolves. Gently fold in the sour cream. Add the pineapple with its juice and stir well. Add the yogurt, cherries, and nuts. Pour into a 9-by-13-inch pan.
2. Refrigerate for 4 to 5 hours, or until firm.

YIELD: 12 SERVINGS          2.5 G FAT                 77 MG SODIUM
SERVING SIZE: 3 INCHES      1.6 G PROTEIN
   BY 4 INCHES              11 G CARBOHYDRATES
CALORIES: 72

# Sunshine Citrus Mold

*A refreshing salad that is great with a meal.*

1 cup boiling water

1 0.3-ounce package sugar-free
lime gelatin

1 0.3-ounce package sugar-free
lemon gelatin

12 ounces sugar-free lemon-lime
soda or ginger ale

8 ounces canned crushed pineapple
(in its own juice)

15 ounces canned mandarin oranges,
drained and rinsed

1/2 cup chopped pecans

1. In a bowl, pour the water over the gelatins and stir until the gelatins dissolve. Add the soda, pineapple, and oranges. Mix well. Add the chopped pecans. Pour into a large mold or a 9-by-13-inch pan.
2. Refrigerate for 4 hours, or until firm.

YIELD: 12 SERVINGS      1 G FAT      64 MG SODIUM
SERVING SIZE: 3 INCHES    1.7 G PROTEIN
   BY 4 INCHES          8.3 G CARBOHYDRATES
CALORIES: 48

# Sparkling White Grape Salad

*A tasty summer salad with a
nice blend of sparkling tartness.*

³/4 cup boiling water

2 0.3-ounce packages sugar-free
sparkling white grape gelatin

12 ounces sugar-free ginger ale or club soda

1 cup natural white grape juice

8 ounces canned crushed pineapple
(in its own juice)

15 ounces canned lite pears,
drained and diced

1. In a bowl, pour the water over the gelatin and stir until the gelatin dissolves. Add the soda and stir again. Stir in the grape juice, pineapple, and pears. Blend well. Pour into a 9-by-13-inch pan.
2. Refrigerate for 4 hours, or until firm.

YIELD: 12 SERVINGS      1 G FAT      70 MG SODIUM
SERVING SIZE: 3 INCHES      1.7 G PROTEIN
     BY 4 INCHES      8 G CARBOHYDRATES
CALORIES: 60

# Pavlova

3 egg whites

¼ teaspoon cream of tartar

⅛ cup sugar

Acesulfame K sugar substitute
equivalent to ¼ cup sugar

1 teaspoon vanilla extract

½ cup 2% milk

⅛ cup ice water

1½ cups crushed strawberries,
unsweetened fresh or frozen

1 cup kiwi slices

1. Preheat oven to 250°. Line a baking sheet with parchment
paper.
2. In a large bowl using an electric mixer at high speed, beat
the egg whites and cream of tartar until peaks form. Gradually add the sugar, sugar substitute, and vanilla. Spread the
meringue on the parchment paper to form an 8-by-12-inch
rectangle with raised sides.
3. Bake for 1 hour, or until firm. Turn off oven. Cool in the
oven for 2 hours, without opening the door.
4. In a chilled medium bowl using an electric mixer, beat the
milk and water until peaks form. Spread over the meringue.
Spoon the strawberries and kiwi over the top before serving.

YIELD: 8 SERVINGS
SERVING SIZE: 1 INCH
   BY 1½ INCHES
CALORIES: 75

0 G FAT
2 G PROTEIN
17 G CARBOHYDRATES

25 MG SODIUM
200 MG POTASSIUM

# Chilled Fruit Mix

20 ounces canned pineapple chunks
(in its own juice)

2 oranges, peeled and sectioned

2 kiwi fruit, peeled and sliced

1 pear, peeled and sliced

¼ cup ground ginger

fresh mint, for garnish

1. Drain the pineapple, reserving ½ cup juice. In a large bowl, combine the pineapple, oranges, kiwi, and pear. Add the ginger to the reserved pineapple juice. Pour over the fruit.
2. Refrigerate for 2 to 3 hours, stirring 2 or 3 times to mingle flavors. Garnish with a sprig of fresh mint before serving.

YIELD: 4 SERVINGS
SERVING SIZE: ½ CUP
CALORIES: 88
EXCHANGES: 2 FRUIT

# Fresh Fruit Compote

*A very attractive dessert,*
*best served in a glass bowl.*

3 pears, peeled and cubed

3 tablespoons lemon juice

1 large orange, peeled and sectioned

1 small honeydew, peeled and cubed

1/2 pound seedless red grapes

1/2 cup water

3 packets Acesulfame K sugar substitute

1/4 teaspoon nutmeg

1. Sprinkle the pears with 1 tablespoon of the lemon juice. In a large bowl, combine the fruit. In a small bowl, stir together the remaining lemon juice with the water, sugar substitute, and nutmeg. Pour over the fruit.
2. Refrigerate for 2 hours before serving.

YIELD: 8 SERVINGS                    3 G FIBER                    8 MG SODIUM
SERVING SIZE: 1/2 CUP
CALORIES: 78
EXCHANGES: 1 FRUIT

# Baked Apple

   1 medium apple, cored
     non-stick vegetable cooking spray
 1/2 teaspoon cinnamon
   1 packet Acesulfame K sugar substitute

1. Preheat oven to 375°.
2. Place apple in a baking dish lightly coated with non-stick cooking spray. Apple can be left whole or sliced. Sprinkle with cinnamon and sugar substitute. Cover with aluminum foil.
3. Bake for 45 to 50 minutes.

YIELD: 1 SERVING
CALORIES: 65
EXCHANGES: 1 FRUIT

# Fruit Gelatin

*Remember, gelatin is a free food.*

Add 1 cup fruit to a 0.3-ounce package of gelatin and the entire mixture equals 2 fruit exchanges, or 1/2 fruit exchange for each 1/2 cup serving.

YIELD: 2 CUPS
SERVING SIZE: 1/2 CUP
CALORIES: 32
EXCHANGES: 1/2 FRUIT

1 G FAT
2 G PROTEIN
6 G CARBOHYDRATES

# Lime Gelatin with Blueberries and Peaches

꒰ꔫ꒱

2 0.3-ounce packages sugar-free
  lime gelatin

1 cup boiling water

1 cup cold water

2 cups unsweetened blueberries,
  fresh or frozen

2 cups peeled and sliced peaches,
  fresh or unsweetened frozen

1. In a large bowl, mix the gelatin and boiling water, stirring until well dissolved. Add the cold water and stir again. Add the blueberries and peaches and mix well. Pour into a 9-by-13-inch pan or a 2½-quart mold.

2. Refrigerate for 3 to 4 hours, or until set.

YIELD: 12 SERVINGS          0.7 G PROTEIN               40 MG SODIUM
SERVING SIZE: 3 INCHES      10 G CARBOHYDRATES
   BY 3 INCHES
CALORIES: 5

# Tropicale Dessert

1 banana, sliced

½ cup sliced strawberries

1 drop red food coloring

2 cups honeydew balls

2 cups watermelon balls

4 whole strawberries for garnish

1. Place the banana and strawberries in a blender. Add food coloring. Process until smooth. Cover and refrigerate for one hour.
2. Just before serving, place honeydew balls and watermelon balls into four individual serving dishes. Spoon sauce over melon balls. Garnish with a whole strawberry.

YIELD: 4 SERVINGS     0.05 G FAT     13 MG SODIUM
SERVING SIZE: 1¼ CUPS     1.5 G PROTEIN
CALORIES: 121     25 G CARBOHYDRATES

# Ambrosia

2 oranges, peeled, with pith and
   seeds removed

2 bananas, peeled

2 packets Acesulfame K sugar substitute

¼ cup angel flaked coconut

1. Thinly slice the oranges and bananas. In a serving bowl,
   arrange a layer of orange slices. Sprinkle with some of the
   sugar substitute. Place a layer of the bananas over the oranges, and then a layer of coconut. Continue layering the
   fruit, ending with a layer of coconut. Cover with plastic wrap.
2. Refrigerate for 1 to 2 hours before serving.

YIELD: 4 SERVINGS          3 G FIBER          TRACE SODIUM
CALORIES: 85
EXCHANGES: 1½ FRUIT

# Raspberry Swirl

꽃

1 0.3-ounce package sugar-free
  raspberry gelatin

½ cup hot water

10 ounces frozen raspberries,
  no sugar added, partially thawed

6 ounces frozen unsweetened mixed
  fruit punch concentrate, thawed

1½ cups cold water

1 cup low-fat sour cream

1. In a large bowl, combine the gelatin and hot water and stir until dissolved. Drain berries and reserve juice. Stir juice, punch concentrate, and cold water into gelatin.
2. In a small bowl, gently blend 1 cup of the gelatin mixture into the sour cream. Refrigerate both mixtures for 3 to 4 hours, or until set.
3. Fold the berries into the plain gelatin mixture. Layer mixtures in a 2-quart mold. Cut through both to create a swirled effect.
4. Refrigerate for 3 to 4 hours, or until firm.

YIELD: 9 SERVINGS
SERVING SIZE: ¼ CUP
CALORIES: 50
EXCHANGES: ½ FAT; 1 FRUIT

# PUDDINGS

## Tips for Puddings

- To unmold puddings after refrigeration, run a knife around the edge of the dish or mold. Invert over a plate. Place a damp hot cloth over the mold and shake gently to release. Lift the mold.
- Place a piece of wax paper over a hot pudding to avoid getting a "skin" on the top of the pudding.
- When making a custard-style pudding, following directions carefully, as this kind of pudding curdles easily.
- Custard puddings should be cooked or baked on low heat, as high heat causes it to curdle, resulting in a thin, lumpy texture.
- Sweetened condensed milk, with no or low fat, has a thicker consistency. It will not get "sugary" when heated and will not form ice crystals in frozen desserts. It will also thicken without heat when used with an acid food such as lemon, lime, orange, pineapple, or apple or with the juices of these fruits.

# Bread Pudding

1 tablespoon low-fat margarine

1 cup dry bread crumbs

1 ½ cups 2% milk, scalded

2 packets Acesulfame K sugar substitute

1 teaspoon cinnamon

2 tablespoons raisins

2 eggs, beaten

1 teaspoon vanilla extract

½ cup unsweetened applesauce

½ teaspoon nutmeg

1. Preheat oven to 325°. Grease an 8-inch square baking dish.
2. Soak the bread crumbs in the scalded milk for 5 minutes. Add the sugar substitute, cinnamon, raisins, eggs, and vanilla extract and mix well. Pour into prepared baking dish.
3. Bake for 50 to 60 minutes.
4. To make the topping, in a saucepan, combine the applesauce and nutmeg. Heat until warm. Pour over cooked bread pudding before serving. Serve warm.

YIELD: 8 SERVING    4 G FAT    145 MG SODIUM
SERVING SIZE: ½ CUP    7.2 G PROTEIN
CALORIES: 130    18 G CARBOHYDRATES

# Pumpkin Custard

15 ounces canned solid-pack pumpkin

2 eggs, beaten

1/3 cup 2% milk

1/8 cup water

1 teaspoon cinnamon

1/2 teaspoon nutmeg

1/2 teaspoon cloves

2 packets Acesulfame K sugar substitute

1. Preheat oven to 325°.
2. In a large bowl, combine the pumpkin, eggs, milk, and water. Beat well. Stir in the spices and sugar substitute. Pour into an 8-inch baking dish.
3. Bake for 35 to 40 minutes, or until tester inserted in the center comes out clean.

YIELD: 4 SERVINGS    3 G FAT    14 G CARBOHYDRATES
SERVING SIZE: 4 INCHES    7 G PROTEIN
   BY 4 INCHES
CALORIES: 103
EXCHANGES: 1/2 MEDIUM MEAT;
   1 STARCH/BREAD

# Rice Pudding

*You'll need the traditional, not the instant,
pudding mix for this savory dessert.*

4 cups 2% milk

1 cup raw quick-cooking rice

¼ cup raisins

1 egg, beaten

2 ounces sugar-free vanilla
  pudding (not instant)

¼ teaspoon cinnamon

¼ teaspoon nutmeg

1. In a large saucepan over medium heat, combine the milk,
   rice, raisins, egg, and pudding mix. Stir until mixture comes
   to a boil. Remove from heat and cool for 5 minutes.
2. Add the cinnamon and nutmeg. Stir well. Serve warm or cool.

YIELD: 8 SERVING
SERVING SIZE: ¾ CUP
CALORIES: 100

2 G FAT
5 G CARBOHYDRATES

# Orange Pudding

¼ cup cornstarch

⅛ cup sugar

3 packets Acesulfame K (or other sugar substitute equivalent to ¼ cup sugar)

¼ teaspoon salt

½ cup unsweetened orange juice

2 eggs

2 cups boiling water

1 tablespoon low-fat margarine

1 teaspoon orange flavoring

grated peel from 1 orange

1 cup non-fat whipped topping (optional)

1. In a medium bowl using an electric mixer at medium speed, combine the cornstarch, sugar, sugar substitute, salt, orange juice, and eggs. Add the boiling water and beat until smooth. Pour mixture into a saucepan and add the margarine.
2. Cook over medium heat for 2 minutes, stirring constantly, until mixture is thickened. Remove from heat, add flavoring and orange peel. Pour ½ cup of pudding into each of six serving dishes.
3. Refrigerate for 30 minutes, or until set. Top with a dollop of whipped topping, if desired, before serving.

YIELD: 3 CUPS
SERVING SIZE: ½ CUP
CALORIES: 100
  (WITHOUT TOPPING)
EXCHANGES: 1 FAT;
  1 STARCH/BREAD

1 G FAT
2 G PROTEIN
15 G CARBOHYDRATES

91 MG CHOLESTEROL

# Raspberry Pudding

1 0.3-ounce package sugar-free
raspberry gelatin

1 cup boiling water

1 cup cold water

1 cup fresh or frozen raspberries

1 ounce instant sugar-free
vanilla pudding mix

1½ cups 2% milk

1 medium banana, sliced

¼ cup flaked coconut

1. Dissolve the gelatin in boiling water. Add the cold water and raspberries. Stir to mix well. Pour into a 9-inch square pan. Refrigerate for 1 hour, or until firm.
2. In a medium bowl, combine the pudding mix and milk. Beat well. Add the banana. Pour pudding over firm gelatin and refrigerate for 3 hours, or until set.
3. Sprinkle coconut over pudding before serving. For extra flavor, toast the coconut before using. To toast coconut, microwave the flaked coconut in a thin layer on a paper plate for four minutes, or until coconut begins to turn light brown, stirring every minute until toasted. (It will continue to brown for one minute after microwaving.)

YIELD: 9 SERVINGS     1 G FAT     1 MG CHOLESTEROL
SERVING SIZE: 3 INCHES     2 G PROTEIN
    BY 3 INCHES     11 G CARBOHYDRATES
CALORIES: 65
EXCHANGES: ¼ FRUIT;
    ⅔ STARCH/BREAD

# Mom's Apple Pudding

❧

*This easy-to-make pudding is an old recipe of
my mother's, which I adapted for a diabetic diet.
Good topped with milk, whipped topping, or
frozen yogurt. Add these calories to total, if used.*

PUDDING:  1 teaspoon low-fat margarine

6 Ida Red or Cortland apples, sliced

1 teaspoon cinnamon

1/2 teaspoon nutmeg

1/8 cup sugar

Acesulfame K sugar substitute
equivalent to 1/8 cup sugar

TOPPING:  1/2 cup water

1 tablespoon low-fat margarine, melted

1/4 cup sugar

Acesulfame K sugar substitute
equivalent to 1/4 cup sugar

1 cup all-purpose flour

1 teaspoon baking powder

1. Preheat oven to 350°. Grease a 2-quart baking dish with
   1 teaspoon margarine.
2. Spread the apples into the prepared dish. Sprinkle with
   the cinnamon, nutmeg, 1/8 cup sugar, and sugar substitute.
   Pour over the apples.
3. In a small bowl, combine the water, melted margarine, 1/4 cup
   sugar, 1/4 cup sugar substitute, flour, and baking powder.
4. Bake for 45 to 50 minutes, or until top is lightly browned
   and apples are soft when pierced with a tester.

YIELD: 8 SERVINGS    5 G FAT
SERVING SIZE: 3/4 CUP    2 G CARBOHYDRATES
CALORIES: 105

# Pistachio Pineapple Pudding

> 1 ounce instant sugar-free
> pistachio pudding mix
>
> 16 ounces canned unsweetened
> crushed pineapple (in its own juice)
>
> ½ cup chopped pecans
>
> 1 cup non-fat whipped topping

1. In a medium bowl, combine the pudding mix, pineapple, pecans, and whipped topping. Stir until well mixed. Pour into a mold.
2. Refrigerate for 3 hours, or until firm.

YIELD: 8 SERVINGS      6 G CARBOHYDRATES      165 MG SODIUM
SERVING SIZE: ½ CUP
CALORIES: 132

# Orange Rice Casserole Dessert

※

*A few drops of lemon juice added to
rice will keep the grains from sticking.*

non-stick vegetable cooking spray

1²/₃ cups 2% milk

3 large eggs

¹/₂ cup sugar

¹/₃ cup raw instant rice

1 teaspoon vanilla extract

1 teaspoon orange extract

¹/₂ teaspoon grated orange peel

dash of salt

dash of nutmeg

1. Preheat oven to 350°. Coat a 2-quart baking dish with non-stick cooking spray.
2. In a small saucepan, heat the milk until hot, but do not boil. In a medium bowl, beat the eggs. Stir in the sugar, rice, vanilla and orange extracts, orange peel, and salt. Stir in the hot milk. Pour into the prepared baking dish. Place the dish in a larger baking pan. Fill the larger pan with boiling water to one inch.
3. Bake for 10 minutes, stir, bake for 10 minutes longer, and stir again. Sprinkle with the nutmeg. Bake for 15 minutes longer, or until a tester inserted in the center comes out clean. Cool on rack for 30 minutes.
4. Refrigerate for 1¹/₂ hours before serving.

| | | |
|---|---|---|
| YIELD: 4 SERVINGS | 3.5 G FAT | 135 MG SODIUM |
| SERVING SIZE: 1 CUP | 6.8 G PROTEIN | 166 MG CHOLESTEROL |
| CALORIES: 180 | 30 G CARBOHYDRATES | |

# Frozen Desserts

## Giving Frozen Desserts Flavor and Texture

Sugar and milk fat give flavor and texture to frozen desserts. When substituting these ingredients, you will have to find a formula that meets your needs.

Artificial sweeteners can be used as a substitute for sugar. Add them to mixtures at room temperature and mix thoroughly until dissolved.

1 packet of artificial sweetener is equivalent to 2 teaspoons of sugar

6 packets equals ¼ cup

Ripeness and sweetness of fruit or juice has an impact on the taste of frozen desserts. You can omit sugar if fruit is extremely ripe or add if fruit is tart. Remember, after freezing, the dessert will taste less sweet than the unfrozen mixture.

The richer the cream you use, the richer the ice cream will be. However, it will have a higher fat content as well.

Heavy cream is the richest with about 35 percent fat. Whipping cream, coffee creamers, and half-and-half contain 30 percent, 18 percent, and 10 percent, respectively.

Milk can also be used as a cream substitute, but the taste and texture will change. I like to use a fat-free sweetened condensed milk, as it improves the taste and also decreases the fat content.

When you are making a frozen ice cream or yogurt, always pre-chill the milk for best results.

| Product | Calories | Fat Content |
| --- | --- | --- |
| 8 ounces heavy cream | 820 | 88 grams |
| 8 ounces half-and-half | 300 | 26 grams |
| 8 ounces 2% milk | 130 | 5 grams |
| 8 ounces 1% milk | 130 | 3 grams |

Long storage of ice cream yogurt should be done in airtight containers.

Ice creams that do not require cooking are best made in an electric mixer, which allows the mixture to increase in volume and become lighter in texture.

# Strawberry Parfait

1 cup all-purpose flour

¼ cup brown sugar

½ cup chopped pecans

¼ cup low-fat margarine

2 egg whites

⅓ scant cup sugar

Acesulfame K sugar substitute
equivalent to ⅓ cup sugar

2 tablespoons lemon juice

2 cups strawberries, hulled and crushed

1 cup non-fat whipped topping

1. Preheat oven to 350°.
2. In a medium bowl, mix together the flour, brown sugar, nuts, and margarine. Reserve ⅓ for topping. Press the remaining ⅔ into a 9-by-13-inch cake pan.
3. Bake for 15 to 20 minutes, or until lightly browned.
4. Meanwhile, in a large bowl using an electric mixer, beat the egg whites until stiff. Add the sugar, sugar substitute, and lemon juice and continue beating constantly until firm. Fold in the strawberries and whipped topping. Spoon into cooled crust. Top with reserved crumbs.
5. Freeze for 3 to 4 hours, or until firm.

YIELD: 20 SERVINGS     3 G FAT     10 MG SODIUM
SERVING SIZE: 2¼ INCHES     0.7 G PROTEIN
    BY 2 INCHES     5 G CARBOHYDRATES
CALORIES: 85

# Fresh Fruit Trifle

*High in calories, but great for a special occasion.
Purchase a pound cake or make one from a package or
your favorite recipe as the basis of this fancy concoction.*

1 pound cake, thinly sliced

2½ teaspoons sherry extract

1 ounce instant sugar-free
vanilla pudding mix

1½ cups 2% milk

1 cup sliced strawberries

½ cup non-fat whipped topping

1. Line the bottom and sides of a 6-cup glass bowl with the cake slices. Sprinkle with 2 teaspoons of the sherry extract.
2. In a medium bowl, combine the pudding mix, milk, and remaining sherry extract. Stir until well blended. Pour over the cake slices. Top with the strawberries. Spread whipped topping over the top.
3. Refrigerate for 4 hours. Garnish with additional fruit if desired.

YIELD: 6 SERVINGS
SERVING SIZE: ⅙ CAKE
CALORIES: 520
EXCHANGES: 3½ FAT;
   1 MILK (2%);
   3 STARCH/BREAD

29 G FAT
2 G FIBER
8 G PROTEIN
57 G CARBOHYDRATES

384 MG SODIUM
250 MG POTASSIUM
46 MG CHOLESTEROL

# Frozen Raspberry Dessert

*This may be frozen in a bowl or poured into a deep-dish prepared pie crust and then frozen, to be served as a frozen pie. Remove from freezer 30 minutes before serving. Remember to add the crust to the nutritional values if you make this as a pie.*

2 0.3-ounce packages sugar-free
  raspberry gelatin

1½ cups boiling water

1 cup cold water

6 ounces non-fat red raspberry yogurt

1 cup non-fat whipped topping

2½ cups fresh or frozen red raspberries
  (no sugar added)

1. In a large bowl, mix the gelatin with the boiling water and stir until dissolved. Add the cold water and continue stirring until well mixed. Refrigerate for 20 minutes.
2. In a small bowl, mix the whipped topping and raspberry yogurt until well blended. Add the topping mixture to the gelatin mixture. Fold in the raspberries and blend well.
3. Freeze for 1 hour, or until firm.

YIELD: 8 SERVINGS       2 G FAT              35 MG SODIUM
SERVING SIZE: ⅛ RECIPE  6 G PROTEIN          210 MG POTASSIUM
CALORIES: 170           22 G CARBOHYDRATES   12 MG CHOLESTEROL

# Blueberry Lime Dessert

*A different but surprisingly good taste sensation.*

2 0.3-ounce packages sugar-free lime gelatin

2 cups boiling water

2 cups cold water

1 8-inch angel food cake

3 cups fresh or frozen blueberries

1 tablespoon fresh lemon juice

1 ounce instant sugar-free vanilla pudding mix

2½ cups 2% milk

2 cups non-fat whipped topping

1. In a medium bowl, combine the gelatin and boiling water and stir until dissolved. Add the cold water and continue stirring until well mixed. Refrigerate until syrupy.
2. Break angel food cake into pieces and line the bottom of a 9-by-13-inch cake pan with them. Add blueberries to syrupy gelatin and stir in the lemon juice. Pour over cake pieces. Refrigerate for 30 minutes, or until firm.
3. In another medium bowl, combine pudding and milk and blend well. Spread pudding on top of gelatin and blueberry mixture.
4. Refrigerate for 3 to 4 hours. Top with whipped topping before serving.

YIELD: 12 SERVINGS
SERVING SIZE: 3 INCHES BY 3¼ INCHES
CALORIES: 180
EXCHANGES: ½ FAT; 1 FRUIT; 1 STARCH/BREAD

# Pronto Frozen Orange Ice

1 0.3-ounce package sugar-free
  orange gelatin
½ cup hot water
1 cup unsweetened, pulp-free
  orange juice

1. In a measuring cup, dissolve the gelatin in the water. Stir in the juice. Pour into a shallow container and freeze for 1 hour, or until slushy. Transfer to a mixing bowl and beat with an electric mixer on high speed until fluffy.
2. Cover and freeze for 2 hours or until firm. Soften slightly before serving.

YIELD: 4 SERVINGS
SERVING SIZE: ½ CUP
CALORIES: 40
EXCHANGES: 1 FRUIT

# Peppermint Ice Cream

*Candy canes give this ice delight a cool, refreshing taste.*

4 eggs

1/3 cup sugar

5 packets Acesulfame K sugar substitute

1/4 teaspoon salt

1 14-ounce can low-fat sweetened condensed milk, chilled

4 cups 2% milk

1/2 teaspoon vanilla extract

1/3 cup crushed hard peppermint candy

1. In a large bowl using an electric mixer, beat the eggs, sugar, sugar substitute, salt, and milks until frothy. Add the vanilla extract and candy, and stir until well blended.
2. Transfer to an ice cream maker and follow directions for freezing.

YIELD: 2½ QUARTS;
   12 SERVINGS
SERVING SIZE: ¾ CUP
CALORIES: 165

1.8 G FAT
2.5 G PROTEIN
20 G CARBOHYDRATES

45 MG SODIUM
0.6 MG CHOLESTEROL

# Kiwi Sorbet

    1 cup boiling water

    ¼ cup sugar

    7 packets Acesulfame K sugar substitute

    4 teaspoons lemon juice

    5 kiwi fruit, peeled and sliced

1. In a small saucepan, combine the water, sugar, and sugar substitute, stirring until the sugars dissolve. Pour into a large bowl. Refrigerate for 20 minutes.
2. When chilled, add the juice.
3. Place the kiwi in a blender and process until smooth. Stir into the sugar mixture. Pour into an 8-inch square pan. Freeze for 1 hour, or until firm.
4. Remove from freezer and break into pieces. Place in a chilled bowl. Using an electric mixer, beat for approximately 5 minutes, or until light and fluffy.
5. Freeze for 3 to 4 hours, or until firm.

YIELD: 6 SERVINGS      15 G CARBOHYDRATES    HIGH IN POTASSIUM
SERVING SIZE: ½ CUP
CALORIES: 60

# Cherry Freeze

16 ounces frozen dark sweet cherries,
pitted (about 4 cups)

4 tablespoons confectioners' sugar

²/₃ cup 2% milk

½ teaspoon almond extract

½ teaspoon vanilla extract

1 14-ounce can non-fat sweetened
condensed milk

1. Place the cherries in a blender and process until chopped finely. With the blender running, add the confectioners' sugar, milk, almond extract, vanilla extract, and condensed milk. Process until well blended and creamy. Pour mixture into a freezer container. Cover with plastic wrap.

2. Freeze for 1½ to 2 hours, or until the consistency of ice cream. Stir before serving.

YIELD: 3 CUPS          3.7 G PROTEIN          11 MG SODIUM
SERVING SIZE: ½ CUP    18 G CARBOHYDRATES     10.5 MG CHOLESTEROL
CALORIES: 111

# Frozen Fruit Dessert with Coconut Crust

*Because this may be prepared ahead and frozen for up to two weeks, it is an ideal party dessert.*

non-stick vegetable cooking spray

3½ ounces flaked coconut

3 tablespoons low-fat margarine, melted

16 ounces canned lite fruit cocktail, all natural, well drained

1 14-ounce can non-fat sweetened condensed milk

½ cup miniature marshmallows

½ cup chopped pecans

8 ounces non-fat sour cream

½ cup chopped maraschino cherries

⅛ cup lime juice

½ cup non-fat whipped topping

1. Coat a 9-by-13-inch pan with non-stick cooking spray.
2. In a medium bowl, combine the coconut and margarine and press into prepared pan.
3. In a large bowl, combine fruit cocktail, condensed milk, marshmallows, pecans, sour cream, cherries, and lime juice. Mix well. Fold in the whipped topping. Pour over the crust. Freeze for 6 to 8 hours, or until firm.
4. Remove from freezer and refrigerate for 2 to 3 hours before serving. Garnish with fresh fruit if desired.

YIELD: 15 SERVINGS  
SERVING SIZE: 2½ INCHES BY 3 INCHES  
CALORIES: 138  

3 G FAT  
3 G PROTEIN  
25 G CARBOHYDRATES  

28 MG SODIUM  
5 MG CHOLESTEROL

# Frozen Black Sweet Cherry Pie

❧

*This great hot weather dessert is different and refreshing!*

1 0.3-ounce package sugar-free
 cherry gelatin

½ cup boiling water

8 ounces low-fat black sweet cherry yogurt

1 cup sugar-free black sweet cherry
 frozen yogurt

½ cup non-fat whipped topping

2 cups pitted black sweet cherries,
 fresh (if canned, drain well)

1 8-inch prepared shortbread crust

1. In a large bowl, mix the gelatin in the water until dissolved.
   Add the yogurt and frozen yogurt and blend well. Stir in the
   whipped topping and cherries and blend well. Pour into the
   prepared crust.
2. Freeze for 4 hours.

| | | |
|---|---|---|
| YIELD: 8 SERVINGS | 5 G FAT | 155 MG SODIUM |
| SERVING SIZE: ⅛ PIE | 4 G PROTEIN | 40 MG POTASSIUM |
| CALORIES: 160 | 27 G CARBOHYDRATES | 2 MG CHOLESTEROL |

# Frozen Peppermint Pie

1 ounce instant, sugar-free,
   non-fat vanilla pudding mix

1 1/2 cups 2% milk

1/2 cup crushed hard peppermint candies

1 8-inch prepared shortbread pie crust

1. In a medium bowl using an electric mixer, blend the pudding mix and milk until well mixed. Add the candies and stir until well combined. Pour into the prepared crust.
2. Freeze for 6 to 8 hours before serving.

YIELD: 8 SERVINGS
SERVING SIZE: 1/8 PIE
CALORIES: 137

5 G FAT
2.5 G PROTEIN
16 G CARBOHYDRATES

117 MG SODIUM
4 MG CHOLESTEROL

# Fruit Flavor Freeze

*Refreshing on a hot summer day.*

1 0.3-ounce package sugar-free
    gelatin, any flavor

⅛ cup sugar

Acesulfame K sugar substitute
equivalent to ⅛ cup sugar

1 cup boiling water

1½ cups 2% milk

½ cup non-fat whipped topping, thawed

1. In a large bowl, combine the gelatin, sugar, sugar substitute, and water and stir until dissolved. Stir in the milk. Mixture will appear curdled, but will be smooth when frozen. Pour into a 9-by-13-inch pan and freeze for 1 hour, or until ice crystals form.
2. Spoon mixture into a chilled bowl. Using an electric mixer, beat until smooth. Blend in the whipped topping. Return to the pan.
3. Freeze for 5 hours, or until firm.

YIELD: 12 SERVINGS     0.6 G FAT     37 MG SODIUM
SERVING SIZE: 3 INCHES     1.4 G PROTEIN     3 MG CHOLESTEROL
    BY 4 INCHES     4 G CARBOHYDRATES
CALORIES: 48

# Frozen Vanilla Yogurt

    1 cup non-fat plain yogurt

    7 ounces canned non-fat sweetened condensed milk

    1 cup 2% milk

    ¼ cup sugar

    Acesulfame K sugar substitute equivalent to ⅓ cup sugar

    2 eggs

    1½ teaspoons vanilla extract

1. Place all ingredients in a blender and mix until smooth.
2. Transfer to an electric yogurt maker and follow directions for freezing.

YIELD: 1 QUART      1 G FAT      84 MG SODIUM
SERVING SIZE: ½ CUP      0.35 G PROTEIN      5 MG CHOLESTEROL
CALORIES: 150      0.78 G CARBOHYDRATES

# Frozen Berry Yogurt

*Use your choice of fruit, strawberries,
raspberries, blackberries, and blueberries,
or a mixture for this taste sensation.*

¼ cup sugar

3 packets Acesulfame K sugar
  substitute (or other sugar substitute
  equivalent to ¼ cup sugar)

1 egg

7 ounces canned non-fat sweetened
  condensed milk

1 cup non-fat plain yogurt

½ cup pureed berries

1. Place the sugar, sugar substitute, egg, milk, and yogurt in a
   blender and process until smooth. Add the berries and
   blend well.
2. Transfer to an electric yogurt maker and follow directions
   for freezing.

YIELD: 1 QUART          0.75 G FAT            0.65 MG SODIUM
SERVING SIZE: ½ CUP     0.24 G PROTEIN        3 MG CHOLESTEROL
CALORIES: 120           2.5 G CARBOHYDRATES

# BEVERAGES

## Frozen Fruit Tip

I use frozen fruits for garnishes and make fruit juices into ice cubes. Fruit makes a "nice touch" and does not dilute the punch. Individual fruits are great to freeze. To freeze fruit:

Place washed seedless red or green grapes on a baking sheet and freeze until firm. Place in freezer bags and use as a snack or garnish.

15 grapes = 60 Calories; 15 g Carbohydrates

Place rinsed raspberries on a baking sheet and freeze until firm. Place in freezer bags and use as an easy dessert, in a fruit salad, or as a snack.

1 cup raspberries = 60 Calories; 15 g Carbohydrates

Place cleaned blueberries on a baking sheet and freeze until firm. Place in freezer bags and use in a dessert or as a snack or garnish.

¾ cup blueberries = 60 Calories; 15 g Carbohydrates

# Hawaiian Sunrise Punch

*Serve at a special breakfast, brunch, or luncheon.*
*The grenadine gives a festive "sunrise" effect.*

- 1/4 cup unsweetened orange juice
- 2 tablespoons unsweetened pineapple juice
- 1 tablespoon lemon or lime juice
- 1/3 cup club soda
- 1/2 teaspoon rum extract
- 4 ice cubes
- 1/4 teaspoon grenadine syrup (optional)
- fresh fruit (such as orange slices, whole strawberries, or lemon slices) for garnish

Combine the juices, club soda, and rum extract. Stir well. Pour over the ice. Drop in the grenadine syrup. Garnish with the fresh fruit.

YIELD: 1 SERVING
SERVING SIZE: 1 CUP
CALORIES: 54
EXCHANGES: 1 FRUIT
1 G PROTEIN
13 G CARBOHYDRATES
38 MG SODIUM
180 MG POTASSIUM

# Cranberry Cooler

4 cups (1 quart) cranberry juice
cocktail, unsweetened

1½ cups club soda

Combine the cranberry juice cocktail and club soda. Pour over ice.

YIELD: 5½ CUPS
SERVING SIZE: 1 CUP
CALORIES: FREE
EXCHANGES: 1 FRUIT

# Fruit-Flavored Milk Shake

2 cups 2% cold milk

1 0.3-ounce package sugar-free gelatin,
any flavor

2 cups frozen vanilla yogurt, sugar-free

Pour the milk, gelatin, and yogurt into blender. Blend for one minute. Pour into glasses and serve.

YIELD: 4 SERVINGS         6.6 G FAT                40 MG SODIUM
SERVING SIZE: 1 CUP       4 G PROTEIN
CALORIES: 148             6 G CARBOHYDRATES

# Bride's Punch

*This party beverage makes a wonderful centerpiece when served in a punch bowl garnished with floating fruit rings. For a special treat, add a scoop of frozen yogurt or sherbet to each glass, remembering to include it in the nutritional contents.*

12 ounces frozen unsweetened
    orange juice concentrate, thawed
6 ounces frozen unsweetened
    lemonade concentrate, thawed
2½ cups sugar-free ginger ale
6 cups cold water

Combine the juice concentrates, ginger ale, and water. Mix well.

YIELD: 20 SERVINGS          22 G CARBOHYDRATES
SERVING SIZE: ½ CUP
CALORIES: 80

# Low-Fat Milk Shake

*For easier cleaning of a blender, add a drop*
*of detergent to 1 cup of water and turn it on*
*for a few seconds. Rinse and drain dry.*

1 cup cold water

2 packets Acesulfame K sugar substitute

1 partially frozen banana, sliced

$\frac{1}{8}$ cup frozen strawberries

4 ice cubes

$\frac{1}{2}$ cup 2% milk

Place all ingredients into blender. Blend about 2 minutes, or until the ice is finely crushed. Pour into glasses and serve immediately.

YIELD: 2 SERVINGS
SERVING SIZE: 1 CUP
CALORIES: 105
EXCHANGES: 1 $\frac{1}{2}$ FRUIT; $\frac{1}{2}$ MILK

5 g PROTEIN
18 g CARBOHYDRATES

# Citrus Punch

*This cool, refreshing hot-weather drink
was a favorite at our R&D luncheons.*

6 ounces frozen unsweetened
  orange juice concentrate, thawed

6 ounces frozen unsweetened
  lemonade concentrate, thawed

6 ounces frozen unsweetened
  limeade concentrate, thawed

4 cups cold water

2 liters sugar-free lemon-lime soda,
  chilled

In a large pitcher, combine the juices. Stir until well blended.
Add the water and lemon-lime soda and stir again. Pour into
glasses and serve immediately.

YIELD: 18 SERVINGS
SERVING SIZE: 1/2 CUP
CALORIES: 90

# Party Punch

❧

*I added more ingredients to my Any Color Slush recipe from* The Type II Diabetes Cookbook *to make this delicious party drink.*

6 ounces sugar-free gelatin powder, any flavor

2 cups hot water

1 cup cold water

12 ounces frozen unsweetened lemonade concentrate

2 cups unsweetened pineapple juice

2 liters sugar-free lemon-lime soda

1 quart frozen yogurt or sherbet, sugar-free

Place the gelatin in a bowl. Add the hot water and stir until dissolved. Stir in the cold water, lemonade concentrate, and half the pineapple juice. Freeze until firm. Remove from freezer and pour in the soda. Stir to form a slush. Transfer to a blender. Add the remaining pineapple juice, and frozen yogurt or sherbet and blend until smooth. Pour into glasses and serve immediately.

YIELD: 10 SERVINGS
SERVING SIZE: 1 CUP
CALORIES: 80
EXCHANGES: 1 FAT; 1 FRUIT

# Orange Malt

2 cups low-fat plain yogurt

6 ounces unsweetened frozen
orange juice concentrate, thawed

12 ounces sugar-free orange-flavored
carbonated soda

1 level tablespoon malt powder

1 packet Acesulfame K sugar substitute

Place the yogurt and orange juice concentrate into blender.
Mix well. Add the orange-flavored soda, malt powder, and
sugar substitute and blend well again. Serve in chilled glasses.

YIELD: 4 SERVINGS     2 G FAT     80 MG SODIUM
SERVING SIZE: 1 CUP     7 G PROTEIN
CALORIES: 150     25 G CARBOHYDRATES

# Orange Shake

2¼ cups low-fat frozen orange yogurt

12 ounces sugar-free orange-flavored
carbonated soda

Mix all ingredients in blender. Pour into glasses. Serve
immediately.

YIELD: 4 SERVINGS     3 G FAT     8 MG CHOLESTEROL
SERVING SIZE: 1 CUP     2 G PROTEIN
CALORIES: 120     18 G CARBOHYDRATES

# Lemon and Orange Float

*Delicious on a summer's day.*

- ½ cup sugar-free lemon-flavored ice tea mix
- 1 quart cold water
- 6 ounces frozen orange juice concentrate, thawed, unsweetened
- ½ cup frozen vanilla yogurt

Combine the ice tea mix, water, and juice concentrate. Store in the refrigerator until ready to use. To serve, place 6 ounces of iced tea mixture in a glass. Add ½ cup frozen yogurt and stir well. Refrigerate reserved tea mixture.

YIELD: 4 SERVINGS          2.5 G FAT
SERVING SIZE: 1 CUP        2 G PROTEIN
CALORIES: 110              10 G CARBOHYDRATES

# Banana Whip

❧

1 0.3-ounce package sugar-free gelatin,
   any flavor
¾ cup boiling water
½ cup cold 2% milk
   ice cubes
1 medium banana, sliced

Place the gelatin and boiling water in a blender. Process until dissolved. In a measuring cup, combine the milk and ice cubes to make 1¼ cups. Stir until ice is partially melted. Add the milk mixture and banana and blend until smooth.

YIELD: 5 SERVINGS
SERVING SIZE: ½ CUP
CALORIES: 45
EXCHANGES: FREE FOOD

# BREADS AND MUFFINS

## Citrus Zest Tip

The colorful outermost layer of citrus fruit is full of essential oils that contribute flavor and aroma to many foods. Be sure to thoroughly wash and dry the fruit before grating.

- Use a small sharp hand grater to grate a lemon, lime, or orange.
- Grate only the yellow outer layer of the fruit, called zest. Avoid grating the white layer beneath the zest, called the pith, as it has a bitter flavor.

# Tangerine Bread

✥

2 cups all-purpose flour

2 teaspoons baking powder

1 teaspoon baking soda

½ teaspoon salt

¼ cup sugar

Acesulfame K sugar substitute
equivalent to ¼ cup sugar

1 cup low-fat tangerine yogurt

4 tablespoons low-fat margarine, melted

1 egg

1 tablespoon tangerine peel

1 tangerine, peeled, seeded, and
finely diced in a blender

1. Preheat oven to 375°. Grease a 9-by-5-inch loaf pan with low-fat margarine.

2. In a large bowl, sift together the flour, baking powder, baking soda, salt, sugar, and sugar substitute. In a medium bowl, mix together the yogurt, margarine, egg, and tangerine peel. Mix well. Stir 1 cup of the tangerine into the medium bowl. Add the yogurt mixture to the flour mixture, stirring well to combine. Pour into the prepared pan.

3. Bake for 35 to 40 minutes, or until golden brown and a tester inserted in the center comes out clean. Cool for 5 minutes and transfer to a rack to cool completely. This bread freezes well.

YIELD: 24 PIECES,
⅜-INCH THICK
SERVING SIZE: 1 SLICE
CALORIES: 83

2.5 G FAT
0.3 MG FIBER
2 G PROTEIN
14 G CARBOHYDRATES

115 MG SODIUM
9 MG CHOLESTEROL
4. 5 MG VITAMIN C

# Banana Nut Bread with Yogurt

❧

*You'll need three medium bananas for this*
*quick bread. It works best if they are a bit soft.*

1 teaspoon low-fat margarine

¼ cup low-fat margarine

¼ cup sugar

Acesulfame K sugar substitute
equivalent to ¼ cup sugar

1 egg

1 teaspoon vanilla extract

1 cup complete bran flakes

1½ cups all-purpose flour

2 teaspoons baking powder

½ teaspoon baking soda

½ teaspoon salt

8 ounces low-fat vanilla yogurt

1½ cups mashed banana

½ cup chopped pecans

1. Preheat oven to 350°. Grease a 9-by-5-inch loaf pan.
2. In a large bowl, cream together ¼ cup margarine, sugar, and sugar substitute. Add the egg and vanilla and beat well. In a medium bowl, mix together the bran flakes, flour, baking powder, baking soda, and salt. Add to the large bowl, alternating with the yogurt and mashed banana, mixing well

after each addition. Stir in the pecans and mix well. Pour into the prepared pan.

3. Bake for 55 to 60 minutes, or until a tester inserted in the center comes out clean. Cool for 5 minutes and then transfer to a rack to cool completely. This bread freezes well.

YIELD: 24 SLICES,
⅜-INCH THICK
SERVING SIZE: 1 SLICE
CALORIES: 82
EXCHANGES: 1 FRUIT;
1 STARCH/BREAD

4 G FAT
2 G PROTEIN

86 MG SODIUM
16 G CARBOHYDRATES

# Grape Nuts™ Muffins

❦

*Cereal gives these terrific muffins a delicious nutty taste.*

1½ cups all-purpose flour

1 tablespoon baking powder

½ teaspoon salt

1 egg

1 cup 2% milk

⅓ cup canola oil

⅓ cup brown sugar

brown sugar substitute equivalent
to ⅓ cup brown sugar

½ teaspoon cinnamon

½ teaspoon nutmeg

2 cups Grape Nuts™ cereal

¼ cup chopped pecans or walnuts

1. Preheat oven to 400°. Line muffin tins with paper baking cups.
2. In a large bowl, mix together the flour, baking powder, and salt. In a medium bowl, mix together the egg, milk, oil, brown sugar, brown sugar substitute, and spices. Stir the sugar mixture into the flour mixture until well moistened. Fold in the cereal and nuts. Pour into the prepared tins.
3. Bake for 30 to 35 minutes. Cool on a rack until serving.

| | | |
|---|---|---|
| YIELD: 15 MUFFINS | 8 G FAT | 101 MG SODIUM |
| SERVING SIZE: 1 MUFFIN | 3.5 G PROTEIN | 53 MG POTASSIUM |
| CALORIES: 153 | 20 G CARBOHYDRATES | 1.5 MG CHOLESTEROL |

# Orange Bread

3 cups all-purpose flour

¼ cup sugar

Acesulfame K sugar substitute equivalent to ¼ cup sugar

4 teaspoons baking powder

½ teaspoon salt

1 egg

¼ cup 2% milk

¼ cup unsweetened orange juice

1 tablespoon grated orange peel

8 ounces non-fat orange-flavored yogurt

3 tablespoons low-fat margarine, melted

½ cup chopped walnuts

1. Preheat oven to 350°.
2. In a large bowl, sift together the flour, sugar, sugar substitute, baking powder, and salt. Add the egg, milk, orange juice, orange peel, yogurt, and margarine. Mix until well blended. Add the nuts and mix well. Pour into greased 9-by-5-inch loaf pan.
3. Bake for 50 to 60 minutes, or until a tester inserted in the center comes out clean. Cool on a rack before serving.

YIELD: 12 SLICES, ¾-INCH THICK
SERVING SIZE: 1 SLICE
CALORIES: 96
EXCHANGES: 1 FAT; 1 FRUIT; 1 STARCH/BREAD

# Strawberry Bread

3 cups mashed strawberries, unsweetened

3 cups all-purpose flour

1 teaspoon baking powder

1 teaspoon cinnamon

1 teaspoon salt

⅛ cup sugar

Acesulfame K sugar substitute
equivalent to ¾ cup sugar

1¼ cups vegetable oil

4 eggs, well beaten

2 drops red food coloring


TOPPING:  1 packet Acesulfame K
sugar substitute

3 tablespoons all-purpose flour

2 tablespoons low-fat margarine,
melted

1. Preheat oven to 350°. Grease two 9-by-5-inch loaf pans.
2. Drain ½ cup juice from the strawberries and reserve. In a large bowl, mix together the flour, baking powder, cinnamon, salt, sugar, and sugar substitute. Make a well in the center of the mixture. By hand, stir in the oil, eggs, strawberries, and food coloring. Pour into the prepared pans.

3. Bake for 1 hour. Remove from oven. Drizzle the reserved strawberry juice over the breads, return to oven, and bake for another 15 minutes.
4. Cool on a rack. In a small bowl, combine the sugar substitute, flour, and margarine. Drizzle over the top of the breads before serving.

YIELD: 16 SLICES, ½-INCH THICK
SERVING SIZE: 1 SLICE
EXCHANGES: 1½ FAT; 1 FRUIT; 1 STARCH/BREAD

# Applesauce Banana Muffins

*Two medium bananas mashed to yield the ¾ cup
needed to give these muffins their rich taste.*

non-stick vegetable cooking spray

2 cups all-purpose flour

1 ½ teaspoons baking powder

½ teaspoon baking soda

1 teaspoon cinnamon

¼ teaspoon salt

3 packets Acesulfame K sugar substitute

2 eggs

1 teaspoon vanilla extract

1 cup unsweetened applesauce

¾ cup mashed banana

3 tablespoons canola oil

1. Preheat oven to 400°. Spray muffin pans with the non-stick cooking spray or line muffin tins with paper baking cups.
2. In a large bowl, stir together the flour, baking powder, baking soda, cinnamon, salt, and sugar substitute. Add the eggs, vanilla, and applesauce. Beat well. Add the bananas and oil. Stir until well moistened. Pour into the prepared tins.
3. Bake for 20 minutes, or until golden brown. Cool on a rack until serving.

YIELD: 18 MUFFINS     2.5 G FAT     50 MG SODIUM
SERVING SIZE: 1 MUFFIN     2 G PROTEIN     10 MG CHOLESTEROL
CALORIES: 62

# Lemon Yogurt Poppyseed Bread

*This interesting bread is filled with the
refreshing flavor of citrus and poppyseeds.*

2½ cups all-purpose flour

⅓ cup sugar

Acesulfame K sugar substitute
equivalent to ⅓ cup sugar

1 teaspoon baking powder

½ teaspoon baking soda

½ teaspoon salt

2 tablespoons lemon juice

1 teaspoon grated lemon peel

1 teaspoon lemon extract

8 ounces low-fat lemon yogurt

2 eggs

⅛ cup 2% milk

1 teaspoon poppy seeds

1. Preheat oven to 350°.
2. In a large bowl, mix together the flour, sugar, sugar substitute, baking powder, baking soda, and salt. Stir in the lemon juice, lemon peel, and lemon extract. Blend in the yogurt, eggs, and milk, and mix well. Add the poppyseeds and mix until well blended. Pour batter into a 9-by-5-inch loaf pan.
3. Bake for 55 to 60 minutes, or until a tester inserted in the center comes out clean. Cool for 5 minutes, then transfer to a rack to cool completely. This bread freezes well.

YIELD: 24 SLICES,          2 G FAT               62 MG SODIUM
   ⅜-INCH THICK          2 G PROTEIN          6 MG CHOLESTEROL
SERVING SIZE: 1 SLICE    14 G CARBOHYDRATES
CALORIES: 65

# Pear Bran Bread

❧

*A favorite at our R&D meals, this bread has a
delightfully different taste that goes great with salads
and is also very good served with cream cheese or preserves.*

non-stick vegetable cooking spray

1 1/2 cups all-purpose flour

1/4 cup granulated sugar

3 packets Acesulfame K sugar substitute

brown sugar substitute
equivalent to 1/8 cup brown sugar

1 teaspoon cinnamon

1/4 teaspoon nutmeg

1/2 teaspoon baking soda

1/4 teaspoon baking powder

2 eggs

1/4 cup vegetable oil

1/2 teaspoon orange extract

2 tablespoons unsweetened orange or
orange-pineapple juice

15 ounces canned all natural pears, chopped
(makes 3/4 cup), or 1 large pear, chopped

3/4 cup bran flakes

1/8 cup chopped pecans

1. Preheat oven to 350°. Coat a 9-by-5-inch loaf pan with non-stick vegetable cooking spray.
2. In a large bowl, stir together the flour, sugar, sugar substitutes, cinnamon, nutmeg, baking soda, and baking powder.

In a small bowl, combine the eggs, oil, orange extract, and orange juice. Add the egg mixture to the flour mixture, stirring until moistened. The batter will be stiff. Stir in the pears and bran flakes until well mixed. Blend in the pecans. Pour into the prepared pan.

3. Bake for 50 to 60 minutes, or until a tester inserted in the center comes out clean. Cool on a rack until serving.

YIELD: 16 SLICES,
 ½-INCH THICK
SERVING SIZE: 1 SLICE
CALORIES: 110

4 G FAT
1 G FIBER
2 G PROTEIN

50 MG SODIUM
50 MG POTASSIUM
19 G CARBOHYDRATES

# Peach Bread

*This peachy bread is definitely delightful! While fresh peaches are best, you can also use peaches canned in water.*

non-stick vegetable cooking spray

$^1/_2$ cup low-fat margarine

$^1/_3$ cup granulated sugar

Acesulfame K sugar substitute equivalent to $^1/_3$ cup sugar

2 eggs

$^1/_4$ cup low-fat (1% )buttermilk

2 cups all-purpose flour

1 teaspoon baking soda

$^1/_2$ teaspoon salt

2 teaspoons lemon juice

2 cups chopped fresh peaches, or 1 16-ounce can all natural peaches

TOPPING:  1 teaspoon sugar

Acesulfame K sugar substitute equivalent to 1 teaspoon sugar

3 tablespoons all-purpose flour

1 teaspoon cinnamon

2 tablespoons low-fat margarine, melted

1. Preheat oven to 350°. Coat a 9-by-5-inch loaf pan with non-stick cooking spray.

2. In a large bowl, cream the margarine, sugar, and sugar substitute until light and fluffy. Add the eggs and buttermilk and beat thoroughly. Add the flour, baking soda, and salt and beat well. Stir in the lemon juice and peaches and mix well. Pour into the prepared pan. In a small bowl, mix together the topping ingredients. Sprinkle over the bread dough.

3. Bake for 1 hour, or until a tester inserted in the center comes out clean. Cool on a rack until serving.

YIELD: 16 SLICES,
½-INCH THICK
SERVING SIZE: 1 SLICE
CALORIES: 74

1 G FAT
14 G CARBOHYDRATES

10 MG SODIUM
105 MG POTASSIUM

# Orange Applesauce Muffins

*These moist morsels will quickly become
a favorite, both in taste and texture.*

2 cups all-purpose flour

1½ teaspoons baking powder

½ teaspoon baking soda

1 teaspoon cinnamon

¼ teaspoon salt

3 packets Acesulfame K sugar substitute

1 egg

1 cup unsweetened applesauce

1 teaspoon grated orange peel

½ cup unsweetened orange juice

3 tablespoons canola oil

1. Preheat oven to 400°. Line muffin tins with paper baking cups.
2. In a large bowl, stir together the flour, baking powder, baking soda, cinnamon, salt, and sugar substitute. Add the egg, applesauce, orange peel, orange juice, and canola oil. Stir until well moistened. Pour into the prepared tins.
3. Bake for 20 minutes, or until golden brown. Cool on a rack until serving.

YIELD: 18 MUFFINS    3 G FAT    54 MG SODIUM
SERVING SIZE: 1 MUFFIN    2 G PROTEIN    12 MG CHOLESTEROL
CALORIES: 82

# Bran Muffins

1 cup bran flakes

1 cup low-fat sour milk

1 egg

⅓ cup canola oil

1 cup all-purpose flour

1½ teaspoons baking soda

brown sugar substitute
equivalent to ¼ cup brown sugar

¼ cup raisins (optional)

1. Preheat oven to 350°. Line muffin tins with paper baking cups.
2. In a large bowl, combine the bran and sour milk. Let stand about 5 minutes, or until the bran flakes soak up most of the milk. Add the egg and oil and beat well. In a medium bowl, sift together the flour, baking soda, and sugar substitute. Add to the bran mixture and stir until well combined. Add the raisins, if using. Pour into muffin tins.
3. Bake for 25 minutes, or until browned. Cool on a rack until serving.

YIELD: 10 MUFFINS
SERVING SIZE: 1 MUFFIN
CALORIES: PLAIN—143;
      WITH RAISINS—154
EXCHANGES: PLAIN—1½ FAT; 1 STARCH/BREAD;
      WITH RAISINS—1½ FAT; ½ FRUIT; 1 STARCH/BREAD

# Savory Snacks, Sauces, and Vegetable Salads

## Edible Fresh Herbs and Flowers

Many herbs and flowers are edible. They make a simple dessert look elegant, giving an everyday meal a fabulous finish. Use herbs in salads and breads. Use flowers to garnish breads, salads, and desserts. Colorful, edible herbs and flowers also make an attractive addition to the plate. Some suggestions are:

| Herbs | Flowers |
|---|---|
| Basil | Calendula |
| Dill | Day lilies |
| Chives | Nasturtiums |
| Fennel | Violets |
| Mint oregano | Hollyhock |
| Summer savory | Rose |
| Lemonbalm | |
| Rosemary | |
| Sweet marjoram | |
| Lavender | |

It is fun to use flower and herb garnishes along with beautiful napkins to make any meal a very festive occasion.

# Cheese Puffs

4 ounces sharp cheddar cheese spread or
$\frac{1}{2}$ cup grated cheddar cheese,
at room temperature

$\frac{1}{2}$ cup low-fat margarine, softened

1 cup all-purpose flour

$\frac{1}{8}$ teaspoon paprika

1. Preheat oven to 350°.
2. In a medium bowl, combine the cheese and margarine and mix well. Blend in the flour. Form into small, walnut-size balls and place on baking sheets. Dust with paprika.
3. Refrigerate until thoroughly chilled, about 3 hours. Bake for 15 minutes, or until the bottoms of the puffs are lightly browned. Serve hot.

YIELD: 42 PUFFS      5.8 G FAT          125 MG SODIUM
SERVING SIZE: 2 PUFFS  1.6 G PROTEIN       2.9 MG CHOLESTEROL
CALORIES: 78        5 G CARBOHYDRATES
EXCHANGES: 1 FAT;
  $\frac{1}{2}$ STARCH/BREAD;

# Nibbles

0.8 ounce buttermilk-style
Ranch dressing mix

⅓ cup vegetable oil

½ teaspoon garlic powder

½ teaspoon onion powder

½ teaspoon dried dill

1 teaspoon basil

24 ounces oyster crackers

In a bowl, blend the dressing mix, oil, and spices. Pour over crackers. Mix thoroughly for 2 to 3 minutes. Serve. To ensure freshness and flavor, store in a glass jar.

YIELD: 24 SERVINGS
SERVING SIZE: 33 CRACKERS
CALORIES: 148
EXCHANGES: 1 FAT; 1 ⅓ STARCH/BREAD

6.3 G FAT
2.8 G PROTEIN

# Sugar-Free Creamy Onion Dip

*Serve with crisp vegetables as a relish tray*
*for a quick appetizer or a side dish.*

2 tablespoons dry onion soup mix
1 cup low-fat dairy sour cream

Stir the onion soup mix into the sour cream. Chill until serving.

YIELD: 16 SERVINGS     1.3 G FAT     96.1 MG SODIUM
SERVING SIZE: 1 TABLESPOON   1.4 G PROTEIN    28.6 MG POTASSIUM
CALORIES: 21     0.8 G CARBOHYDRATES
EXCHANGES: ½ FAT     4 MG CHOLESTEROL

# Cottage Cheese Dip

❧

2 tablespoons 2% milk

½ teaspoon lemon juice

12 ounces low-fat cottage cheese

1 tablespoon dry onion soup mix

Blend the milk and lemon juice into the cottage cheese until smooth. Stir in the onion soup mix. Chill until serving. Serve as a dip for vegetables.

YIELD: 20 SERVINGS
SERVING SIZE: 1 TABLESPOON
CALORIES: 20
EXCHANGES: FREE FOOD

# Pita Bread Wedges

12 ounces pita bread

2 tablespoons low-fat margarine, softened

1 small clove garlic, minced or 5 tablespoons garlic powder

dash of oregano

dash of basil

1 tablespoon grated Parmesan cheese

1. Preheat oven to 400°.
2. Divide each pita in half to form two rounds. In a small bowl, combine the margarine and garlic. Spread on inside surface of rounds. Sprinkle with the oregano, basil, and Parmesan cheese. Cut each into 8 pie-shaped wedges. Place on baking sheet.
3. Bake 5 minutes, or until golden brown.

YIELD: 4 SERVINGS
SERVING SIZE: 2 WEDGES
CALORIES: 100
EXCHANGES: 1 ½ FAT; ½ STARCH/BREAD

# Party Snack Mix

½ cup low-fat margarine

½ teaspoon onion powder

1 teaspoon garlic powder

3 teaspoons Worcestershire sauce

2 cups rice cereal

2 cups corn cereal

2 cups bran cereal

1 cup pretzels

2 cups pecans or walnuts

1. Preheat oven to 250°.
2. In a small bowl, combine the margarine, onion powder, garlic powder, and Worcestershire sauce. In a large bowl, combine the cereals. Pour the margarine mixture over cereal and mix well. Add the pretzels and nuts and mix until well coated. Pour into a 9-by-13-inch pan.
3. Bake for 45 minutes, stirring occasionally. Cool before serving. Store in an airtight container.

YIELD: 9 CUPS      6 G FAT
SERVING SIZE: ½ CUP      1 G PROTEIN
CALORIES: 125      16 G CARBOHYDRATES

# Sugar-and-Spice Grape Garnish

1 egg white

2 tablespoons sugar

Acesulfame K sugar substitute
equivalent to 2 tablespoons sugar

½ teaspoon cinnamon

1 pound green grapes

1. In a small bowl, beat the egg white until frothy. In another bowl, mix the sugar, sugar substitute, and cinnamon.
2. Cut the grapes into clusters of 3 to 4 grapes. Holding the stem, dip the grapes into egg white then roll in sugar mixture.
3. Refrigerate overnight, or until coating is set.

SERVING SIZE: 12 GRAPES
CALORIES: 60
EXCHANGES: 1 FRUIT

# Orange Sauce

*Homemade sauces make a simple dessert into something special. Great over frozen yogurt or any cake.*

2¼ cups water

2 tablespoons cornstarch

2 teaspoons sugar-free dry orange-flavored drink mix

mint sprig and orange slice for garnish (optional)

In a saucepan over medium heat, stir together the cornstarch and water until dissolved. Cook, stirring constantly, until clear. Remove from heat. Add the drink mix. Stir well. Serve over cake, pudding, or frozen yogurt. Garnish with a frozen orange slice and mint sprig for a festive presentation.

To make Lemon Sauce, substitute lemon drink mix for the orange drink mix.

For Cinnamon Sauce, use 1 teaspoon vanilla extract and 1 teaspoon cinnamon in lieu of the drink mix.

YIELD: 8 SERVINGS ·      2 G CARBOHYDRATES
SERVING SIZE: ¼ CUP
CALORIES: 10, WHICH ARE FREE
EXCHANGES: ½ FRUIT

# Vanilla Custard Sauce

*This thick sauce makes a nice topping on
puddings, cake, gelatin desserts, and fresh fruit.*

1 cup 2% milk

3 tablespoons sugar

1 tablespoon plus 1 teaspoon cornstarch

2 large egg yolks, beaten

1 teaspoon vanilla extract

1. In a 2-quart saucepan over medium heat, mix the milk, sugar, and cornstarch until smooth. Bring to a boil, reduce heat to low, and boil for one minute. Remove from heat. Gradually stir about one-third of the hot mixture into the egg yolks.
2. Return the egg mixture to the saucepan. Cook over low heat until thickened; do not boil. Pour into a small bowl and stir in vanilla.
3. Refrigerate for 2 to 3 hours. Whisk before serving.

SERVING SIZE: 2 TABLESPOONS    1.5 G FAT      17.5 MG SODIUM
CALORIES: 50                  1.5 G PROTEIN    65 MG CHOLESTEROL
                         7.5 G CARBOHYDRATES

# Lemon Sauce

2 cups water

2 tablespoons cornstarch

⅛ teaspoon salt

2 tablespoons low-fat margarine

2 tablespoons lemon juice

1 tablespoon grated lemon peel

4 packets Acesulfame K sugar substitute

In a 2-quart saucepan over medium heat, combine the water, cornstarch, and salt and stir until smooth. Cook until clear and thickened. Simmer for 1 minute. Remove from heat. Stir in the margarine until melted. Add the lemon juice, peel, and sugar substitute. Stir to mix well. Serve warm over cake or pudding.

YIELD: 4 SERVINGS
SERVING SIZE: ½ CUP
CALORIES: 38
EXCHANGES: ½ FAT; ½ VEGETABLE

3 G CARBOHYDRATES

# Spinach Salad with Mandarin Oranges

2 cups fresh green spinach,
   torn into pieces

11 ounces canned mandarin oranges,
   drained

¼ pound lean bacon, cooked
   crisp and crumbled

¼ small red onion, sliced into thin rings

DRESSING: ¼ cup white vinegar

1 teaspoon sugar

1 packet Acesulfame K
   sugar substitute

⅔ teaspoon dried mustard

½ teaspoon salt

1 tablespoon lemon juice

½ cup canola oil

1 teaspoon poppy seed

In a large salad bowl, combine the spinach, oranges, bacon, and onion. Mix well. In a small bowl, combine all dressing ingredients and mix well. Pour over prepared salad and toss. Serve immediately.

YIELD: 6 SERVINGS
SERVING SIZE: ½ TO ¾ CUP
CALORIES: 297
DRESSING: FREE FOOD,
  LESS THAN 20 CALORIES
  PER TABLESPOON

8 G FAT
1 G FIBER
7 G PROTEIN

8 MG SODIUM
10 G CARBOHYDRATES

# Asian Slaw with Peanuts

4 cups (about 1 head) sliced cabbage,
green or red

4 green onions, sliced

6 ounces snow peas,
strings removed and sliced
(or 6 ounces frozen peas)

⅓ cup unsalted peanuts

DRESSING: ½ cup vegetable oil

¼ cup rice vinegar

2 tablespoons sesame seed oil

1 tablespoon ginger

2 teaspoons soy sauce

1 teaspoon white pepper

In a large salad bowl, combine all ingredients and mix well. In a medium bowl, mix all the dressing ingredients together. Pour over prepared salad and toss. Serve immediately.

YIELD: 4 SERVINGS     1 G FAT     6 G CARBOHYDRATES
SERVING SIZE: 1 CUP     3 G FIBER
CALORIES: 280     2 G PROTEIN

# Creamy Salad Dressing

1 cup low-fat cottage cheese

2 tablespoons 2% milk

1½ teaspoons dry salad dressing
mix of your choice

In a blender, blend the cottage cheese and milk until smooth.
Add the salad dressing mix. Blend until thoroughly mixed.

YIELD: 8 SERVINGS
SERVING SIZE: 1 TABLESPOON
CALORIES: 30
EXCHANGES: ½ LEAN MEAT

# Yogurt Salad Dressing

*Use this quick mix as a dressing
for greens or a vegetable dip.*

1 envelope ranch dressing mix

1 cup low-fat plain yogurt

1 cup low-fat (1%) buttermilk

1 packet Acesulfame K sugar substitute

In a small bowl, combine all ingredients and mix well.

YIELD: 16 SERVINGS
SERVING SIZE: 1 TABLESPOON
CALORIES: 18

LESS THAN 1 G FAT
1 G PROTEIN
2 G CARBOHYDRATES

# Creamy Lime Dressing

❧

*Use this dressing on a vegetable salad or for greens.*

    1 cup low-fat sour cream
    2 tablespoons lime juice
    1 teaspoon grated lime peel
    1 packet Acesulfame K sugar substitute
      dash of cilantro
      dash of cardamom

In a small bowl, combine all ingredients and mix well.

YIELD: 1 CUP
SERVING SIZE: 1 TABLESPOON
CALORIES: 10
EXCHANGES: FREE FOOD

# Garlic Vinaigrette

*Excellent on Spinach and Rice Salad
and other green salads.*

½ cup vinegar

2 tablespoons vegetable oil

½ teaspoon onion powder

1 teaspoon garlic powder

1 teaspoon celery powder

½ teaspoon paprika

In a jar, combine all ingredients and shake vigorously. Pour over prepared salad.

YIELD: 10 SERVINGS          3.4 G FAT          140 MG SODIUM
SERVING SIZE: 1 TABLESPOON   1 G CARBOHYDRATES
CALORIES: 34

# Cottage Cheese Salad Dressing

    1 cup low-fat cream-style cottage cheese
    ¹/₄ cup water
    1 ¹/₂ tablespoons lemon juice
    2¹/₂ tablespoons chopped dill pickle
    1 tablespoon minced onion

In a blender, puree the cottage cheese, water, and lemon juice until smooth. Stir in the pickle and onion. Refrigerate until serving.

YIELD: 1 CUP
SERVING SIZE: 1 TABLESPOON
CALORIES: 16
EXCHANGES: FREE FOOD

# Vegetable Salad

*Top these greens with any one of the delicious dressings,
just be sure to include the nutritional information.*

1 cup lettuce, cut up

1 tomato, chopped

3 tablespoons chopped celery

2 tablespoons chopped green pepper

1 tablespoon chopped onion

1/4 small cucumber, sliced

1 egg, hard boiled and grated

1/4 cup low-fat Parmesan cheese, grated

In a large salad bowl, combine all ingredients and toss well.

YIELD: 2 SERVINGS      3.7 G FAT
SERVING SIZE: 1 1/2 CUPS      6.2 G PROTEIN
CALORIES: 70      2.5 G CARBOHYDRATES

# Cucumber Salad

½ cup boiling water

1 0.3-ounce package sugar-free lime gelatin

1 tablespoon vinegar

1 medium cucumber, peeled and diced

1 small onion, chopped

½ cup chopped celery

½ cup low-fat mayonnaise

2 cups low-fat cottage cheese

½ cup chopped pecans

5 ounces canned crushed pineapple (in its own juice)

In a large bowl, pour the water over the gelatin and stir until the gelatin dissolves. Add the remaining ingredients and mix well. Pour into a 9-by-13-inch pan. Refrigerate for 4 hours, or until firm.

YIELD: 12 SERVINGS
SERVING SIZE: 3 INCHES BY 4 INCHES
CALORIES: 120

8 G FAT
6 G PROTEIN
8 G CARBOHYDRATES

# APPENDICES

## ❧ Appendix A

# HOLIDAY PLANNING

Holidays are a stressful time for many people and especially for a diabetic. It is hard to stay on your diabetic diet at home, and much harder when you are out and/or are at a party with people saying, "Try this, a little bite won't hurt you." You must remember that a lot of little bites will hurt you, by raising your blood glucose readings.

With careful planning before the holidays, and a little discipline at the event, you can stay healthy all through the year. These ideas will help you to eat right, lessen the stress of eating out, and enjoy the holidays as well as the parties that come with them.

Decide how you want to live your life. If you want a full and healthy life, begin by staying with a healthy meal plan that will let you function well. Take control of your attitude and of your life. Get your blood glucose readings controlled before the holidays. Get involved in activities that you like to do that give you satisfaction. Then try some new things that will be fun.

Once you have your blood glucose readings under control, and are also feeling good about yourself, it is time to start planning your holiday party!

# Timetable

## *One month before your party:*

- Make and freeze: appetizers, breads, sauces, and desserts.

## *Three weeks before your party:*

- Decide on what type of party you want to have: buffet, sit-down dinner, luncheon, cocktail party, etc. If it is to be a sit-down dinner, invite as many as you can sit comfortably. If it is to be a buffet, keep it simple and have eating areas, so that your guests do not have to "juggle plates." If is to be appetizers, punch, breads, and a light menu, make your decision now.

- Make a guest list. Invite your guests and have them RSVP so that you will know how many people will attend your party.

- Think healthy and light. Your diabetes meal plan will fit right in with diets for people who are on low-fat, low-cholesterol, low-sodium, and low-calorie diets. You can plan a meal that will be healthy, taste good, and be attractive.

- When preparing food for your party, use herbs and spices that are salt-free and fat-free cooking methods.

- To add a festive touch to the food, tint it with food coloring or garnish it with seasonal fruits and herbs.

- Make your table attractive by choosing ingredients that are pleasing to the eye and arranged colorfully.

## *Three or four days ahead:*

- Chop and measure foods for sauces, casseroles, and salads and refrigerate in covered containers.

## *Two days ahead:*

- Make molded salads, salad dressings, and desserts. Chop and slice vegetables and fruits and refrigerate in covered containers.

*One day ahead:*
- Remove the frozen food from the freezer that you prepared earlier, and thaw in the refrigerator. Prepare casseroles, vegetables, and salads that may be refrigerated overnight. Finish preparing fruits, and cover tightly with plastic wrap and refrigerate.
- Start to prepare your table, by getting out serving pieces, silver, hot pads, etc.
- Arrange a centerpiece for your table. (You may have already ordered a special one for your party.)

*Day of the party:*
- Garnish desserts, unmold salads, and arrange foods in appropriate serving dishes.
- Finish setting table.

*Right before the party:*
- Cook and heat foods as necessary.
- Arrange foods on the table.
- Get yourself dressed and ready.

## Safe Food Choices for Parties

Serve safe foods and drinks at your party and choose them when you are out. Safe foods include:
- Crackers and cheese in small cubes
- Fresh fruit in small cubes
- Party snack mix
- Popcorn
- Pretzels
- Fresh fruits and vegetables with low-calorie dips
- Low-fat cheeses and meats

- Low-calorie punch and sugar-free soft drinks
- Low-fat gravy and sauces
- Whole grain breads, muffins, and rolls
- Low-fat, low-cholesterol margarine
- Baked, broiled, and grilled meats
- Pasta with light sauces
- Fruit cups and fruit desserts
- Fruit or vegetable salads with low-fat, low-cholesterol dressings
- Frozen yogurts, sherbets, and sorbets
- Low sugar, low-fat, low-cholesterol recipes from this book

### Safe beverages include:
- Sugar-free soft drinks
- Flavored mineral waters without fructose, sugar, or corn syrup on the ingredients label
- Fruit juice spritzer ( half juice, half sugar-free soda)
- Hot spiced apple cider
- Cold apple cider
- Sparkling apple juice
- Beverage recipes from this book

### Risky foods include those that may raise your blood sugar, such as:
- Fried entrees
- Fatty gravy
- Butter
- Creamy dressings that are "regular"
- Natural cheeses
- Candied dishes
- Alcoholic beverages
- Sweets that are high in sugar, cholesterol, and fat

Enjoy your successful party!

## ❧ Appendix B

# How to Lower
# Your Cholesterol

Most of the cholesterol in your blood is made by your liver from the carbohydrates, fats and protein that you eat. It can also come directly from animal products that you eat. You should have no more than 300 mg of cholesterol per day.

Cholesterol is a naturally occurring fatty substance. It has both good and bad effects on your body. On the good side: it helps build and maintain nerve cells and it builds natural hormones. On the bad side: when your body has too much cholesterol, blood vessel walls can thicken and reduce circulation causing strokes and heart attacks.

Low-density lipoprotein (LDL) is called bad cholesterol. They carry a lot of cholesterol and leave fatty deposits on your artery walls.

High density lipoprotein (HDL) is called good cholesterol. They clean the artery walls and remove extra cholesterol from the body, lowering the risk of heart disease.

It is desirable to have low levels of LDL and high levels of HDL. Recommended levels are:

- Total cholesterol: 200 mg/dL or below.
- LDL: 130 mg/dL or below.
- HDL: 45 mg/dL or higher.

Control your cholesterol by:

- Eating right and exercising.
- Reduce the amount of fat you eat. No more than 30 percent of your daily calories should come from fat, and only 10 percent of the fat you eat should be saturated fat.
- Check food labels for nutritional facts and ingredients.
- Some kinds of fats are better than others. Butter, some oils, poultry fat, and some meats contain a lot of saturated fat. Polyunsaturated and monounsaturated fats are better for you. Polyunsaturated fat is found in fish and some vegetable oils. Monounsaturated fats are found in olive oil, canola oil, and avocados.
- Limit the amount of margarine and butter that you eat.
- Remove the skin from chicken.
- Drink low-fat milk.
- Use canola oil, olive oil, soybean oil, sunflower oil, or safflower oil, rather than palm or coconut oil.
- Choose lean cuts of meat. Eat lean chicken, turkey or fish, and less red meat.
- Use salad dressings and margarines made with monounsaturated fat.
- Eat foods with fiber every day, as the fiber reduces cholesterol. High fiber foods include fruits, vegetables, beans, and whole grains.
- Use egg whites rather than whole eggs whenever possible.
- Substitute low-fat yogurt and low-fat cottage cheese for sour cream. If you use sour cream, buy the low-fat or non-fat varieties.
- Exercise helps you keep your weight down and increases your HDL (good cholesterol). Include some aerobic exercise, which keeps your heart rate up. Walking, bicycling, jogging, swimming, stair climbing, and steppers do this. Start an exercise program slowly, with your doctor's approval.

- Use non-stick sprays.
- Bake, grill, microwave, broil, or steam foods.
- Season with herbs, spices, butter-flavored powders, and lite or low-fat dressings.
- When eating out, be assertive. Ask for dressings "on the side" and less cheese and/or mayonnaise on a sandwich and order food that is prepared in healthy ways.
- Stop smoking. Smoking lowers your good cholesterol (HDL) and increases your risk of cancer, heart attack, and stroke. Also, smoking is harmful for a person with diabetes because it can raise blood sugar readings and cause serious health problems in a diabetic.

## ❧ Appendix C

# RECIPE MODIFICATIONS

Don't throw out your favorite recipes. Below is a list of possible low-fat, sodium, and sugar substitutions that can be used to make your recipes healthier. Try adapting some of your old favorites using recipe modifications.

Most important: Be creative and positive and keep repeating the recipe until you "get it right."

| Ingredients | Possible Substitutions |
|---|---|
| Butter, margarine, or cooking oil | The availability of non-stick frying pans makes non-fat cooking possible. Non-stick vegetable cooking sprays work well to prevent sticking. Replace fat with equal amounts of defatted stocks (beef, chicken, or vegetable), wine, juice, water, or other liquids. Fats can be left out of soups, stews, and casseroles. To remove any fat, chill in refrigerator for several hours and remove congealed fat. Each tablespoon of oil eliminated reduces calories by 100. |

| | |
|---|---|
| Cakes, cookies, pastries | Homemade bran muffins or quick bread. Make you own sweet treats by using whole-grain flours, such as oat-meal, and reduce fat. |
| Chocolate | Cocoa or carob, 1 ounce chocolate equals 3 tablespoons cocoa plus 1 table-spoon vegetable oil. Carob powder is low in fat and contains no caffeine. Unsweetened, it is suitable in many recipes. Three to 4 tablespoons carob powder worked into 1 tablespoon non-fat (skim) milk and 1 tablespoon oil is equal to 1 ounce of chocolate. When converting a recipe from chocolate to carob, reduce the amount of sweetener to compensate for carob's natural sweet-ness. Reduce the oven temperature 25° to avoid overbrowning. Avoid carob chips, which contain palm oil, and carob candy bars, which are full of added sugar and fat. |
| Egg (1 whole) | 2 egg whites, or ¼ cup egg substitute. |
| 1 egg yolk | 1 egg white. |
| Light or heavy cream | Replace all or part of the cream with evaporated non-fat (skim) milk. |
| Non-dairy creamer | Evaporated non-fat (skim) milk. |
| Nuts | Raisins. |
| Salad dressing | Standard salad dressing recipes call for a 3:1 ratio of oil to vinegar. This can be easily reduced to 2:1 or 1:1. The ratio will depend on the kind of vinegar used and the other ingredients. Balsamic |

vinegar, a mild Italian vinegar, or rice vinegar need very little oil to produce a tasty dressing.

| | |
|---|---|
| Salt | Reduce to one-half the amount or slightly less in a recipe. Experiment with the use of more herbs and spices to reduce or eliminate salt. Wine, sherry, and low-sodium bouillon add flavor to foods. Prepared mustard and horseradish are excellent flavor additions; use sparingly because they contain some sodium. |
| Sour cream or mayonnaise | Use plain yogurt as a substitute in dips, dressings, desserts, sauces, baking, soups, or marinades. |
| Wheat flour (1 cup) | ¾ cup buckwheat; or ¾ cup coarse cornmeal; or 1 scant cup fine cornmeal; or ¾ cup rye flour; or 1⅓ cups oatmeal. |
| White flour (1 cup all-purpose) | 1 cup whole-wheat flour minus 2 tablespoons; or ½ cup white and ½ cup whole-wheat flour; or ¾ cup white flour and ¼ cup bran. |
| White sauce | Eliminate the fat and blend unbleached flour or cornstarch with non-fat (skim) milk as usual; season to taste. You will reduce calories if you use cornstarch or arrowroot in place of flour; you'll require only about half as much. |
| Whole milk | Non-fat (skim) milk (add extra non-fat dry milk powder to liquid milk for a thicker consistency); you save 72 calories per cup by using non-fat (skim) |

milk. In cooking, 1 cup buttermilk equals 1 cup non-fat milk plus 1 teaspoon lemon juice.

## Baked Goods

There's no need to give up your favorite baked goods to eat leaner. Here's how to reduce the fat in your recipes by one-third to one-half without losing the great taste:

| For a Tasty Dessert | Use This Much Fat |
|---|---|
| Cakes and soft-drop cookies | No more than 2 tablespoons of fat per cup of flour |
| Muffins, quick breads, biscuits | No more than 1 to 2 tablespoons of fat per cup of flour |
| Pie crust | ½ cup margarine for 2 cups flour |
| Sugar | Reduce to ¼ or ½ original amount or use ¼ cup sugar for 1 cup flour |

## Dessert and Beverage Choices

| Instead Of | Choose |
|---|---|
| Apple or cherry pie | Custard or pumpkin pie |
| Candy bar | Ice cream or ice milk |
| Chocolate cake or torte | Angel food or pound cake |
| Cranberry sauce | Cranberries + sugar substitute |
| Fruit canned in sugar syrup | Fruit canned in water or juice |
| Fruit-flavored yogurt | Plain yogurt + sugar substitute |
| Fruit gelatin | Sugar-free gelatin |
| Pancake syrup | Applesauce (unsweetened) |
| Shortening | Non-stick cooking spray or vegetable oil. 1 cup shortening equals ¾ cup vegetable oil |

| Sugar in coffee or tea | Sugar substitute in coffee or tea. 2 teaspoons sugar equals 1 packet Acesulfame K sugar substitute |
| Sweetened soft drinks | Sugar-free soft drinks |

*Source: Memorial Medical Center of West Michigan*

This diagram illustrates the food groups and the key nutrients in each group. Use the diagram to determine your daily food choices. Vegetables are on top and should lead the way. Fats, alcohol, and sweets are on the bottom and provide lots of calories for the few nutrients they contain. In fact, alcohol is truly the "empty" calorie because it robs the body of nutrients and offers none in return.

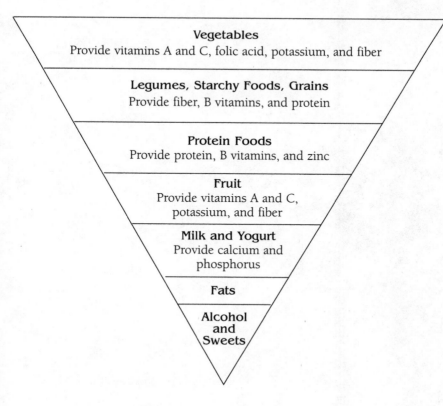

**Vegetables**
Provide vitamins A and C, folic acid, potassium, and fiber

**Legumes, Starchy Foods, Grains**
Provide fiber, B vitamins, and protein

**Protein Foods**
Provide protein, B vitamins, and zinc

**Fruit**
Provide vitamins A and C,
potassium, and fiber

**Milk and Yogurt**
Provide calcium and
phosphorus

**Fats**

**Alcohol
and
Sweets**

# Sugar Substitutions and Artificial Sweetener Equivalencies

## Sugar Substitutes

Remember that sugar adds both crispness and sweetness to a recipe. Sugar helps make baked recipes rise and also taste good. When you substitute for sugar, experiment with a recipe to find a formula that meets your needs.

In the United States, the three major sugar substitutes are: aspartame (Equal™, NutraSweet™, NutraSweet Spoonful™); saccharin (Sweet 'N Low™, Sugar Twin™, Sprinkle Sweet™); and acesulfame K (Sweet One™).

Aspartame must be added after cooking. I prefer acesulfame K for baking and cooking.

### Amount of Artificial Sweeteners to Substitute for Sugar

| Sugar | Acesulfame K | Aspartame | Saccharin |
|---|---|---|---|
| 2 teaspoons | 1 packet | 1 packet | 1 packet |
| 1 tablespoon | 1¼ packets | 1½ packets | 1⅓ packets |
| ¼ cup | 3 packets | 6 packets | 3 packets |
| ⅓ cup | 4 packets | 8 packets | 4 packets |
| 1 cup | 12 packets | 24 packets | 12 packets |

## Sugar Word List

All the below are sugars:

| | |
|---|---|
| Brown sugar | Maltodextrin |
| Corn syrup | Maltose |
| Corn syrup solids | Maple syrup |
| Corn sweeteners | Molasses |
| Crystalline fructose | Natural carbohydrates |
| Dextrose | Raw sugar |
| Fruit sugar | Sorghum |
| High fructose corn syrup | Sucrose |
| Honey | Turbinado |

*Source: Presbyterian Diabetes Center of Albuquerque*

## *Equivalencies for Artificial Sweeteners*

| Sweetener | Amount | Sugar Equivalent |
|---|---|---|
| Sprinkle Sweet™ | 1 teaspoon | 1 teaspoon |
| Sugar Twin™ | 1 teaspoon | 1 teaspoon |
| Sugar Twin™, Brown | 1 teaspoon | 1 teaspoon |
| Sweet 'N Low™ | ¹⁄₁₀ teaspoon | 1 teaspoon |
| | ⅓ teaspoon | 1 tablespoon |
| | 1 teaspoon | ⅙ cup |
| | ½ teaspoon | ¼ cup |
| | 1 tablespoon | ½ cup |
| | 2 tablespoons | 1 cup |
| Adolph's Sugar Substitute™ | 2 shakes of jar | 1 rounded teaspoon |
| | ¼ teaspoon | 1 tablespoon |
| | 1 teaspoon | ¼ cup |
| | 2½ teaspoons | ⅔ cup |
| | 1 tablespoon | ¾ cup |
| | 4 teaspoons | 1 cup |

| Sucaryl™ (liquid sweetener) | ⅛ teaspoon | 1 teaspoon |
|---|---|---|
| | ⅜ teaspoon | 1 tablespoon |
| | ¾ teaspoon | 2 tablespoons |
| | 1½ teaspoons | ¼ cup |
| | 1 tablespoon | ½ cup |
| | 2 tablespoons | 1 cup |
| Weight Watchers Sweet'ner™ | ⅛ teaspoon | 1 teaspoon |
| Sweet 10™, Liquid (6 drops = ⅛ teaspoon) | ⅛ teaspoon | 1 teaspoon |
| | ¼ teaspoon | 1 tablespoon |
| | 1 teaspoon | ¼ cup |
| | 1 tablespoon | ¾ cup |
| | 4 teaspoons | 1 cup |
| Sweet 10™, Tablets | 1 tablet | 1 teaspoon |
| | 3 tablets | 1 tablespoon |
| | 12 tablets | ¼ cup |
| | 36 tablets | ¾ cup |
| | 48 tablets | 1 cup |
| Equal™, Granulated | 1 packet | 2 teaspoons |
| Equal™, Tablets | 1 tablet | 1 teaspoon |

*Prepared by Liz DeShelter, Columbus, Ohio. Reprinted with permission from* Diabetes Care and Education Newsletter, *published by the American Dietetic Association. Consult your nutritionist before using any sweetener.*

# FOOD LISTS

## Milk List

### *Non-Fat (Skim) Milk*

One non-fat choice provides:

    0 g fat

    12 carbohydrates

    8 g protein

    80 calories

Non-fat choices:

    Non-fat (skim) milk

    Powdered, non-fat milk (before adding liquid)

    Sugar-free hot cocoa mix plus 6 ounces water

### *Low-Fat Milk*

One low-fat choice provides:

    3 g fat

    12 g carbohydrates

    8 g protein

    107 calories

Low-fat choices:

    Low-fat (1%) milk

    Yogurt, plain, unflavored, made from non-fat (skim) milk

## Yogurt

Calculate how yogurt fits into the exchange system and the nutritional food values by using the following information:

Non-fat milk      Fat 0 grams; Carbohydrates 12 grams;
                     Protein 8 grams
                     Calories: 90
                     Equal to 1 cup non-fat yogurt
2% milk              Fat 5 grams; Carbohydrates 12 grams;
                     Protein 8 grams
                     Calories: 120
                     Equal to 1 cup plain low-fat yogurt
Whole milk        Fat 8 grams, Carbohydrates 12 grams;
                     Protein 8 grams
                     Calories: 150
                     Equal to 1 cup plain whole milk yogurt

Yogurt is milk to which bacteria have been added to produce lactic acid. Lactic acid gives yogurt a tart taste. Yogurt is an essential part of a low-calorie weight-reduction diet. Your best choice is to buy plain, low-fat yogurt; add sugar substitute and unsweetened fruit.

The varieties of yogurt on the market include original low-fat, non-fat with sugar, non-fat with artificial sweetener, whole milk, non-fat (skim) milk, fruit, custard, fruit on the bottom, and with Swiss cheese. Read labels carefully to be sure of what you are buying. There are also several kinds of frozen yogurt including regular, non-fat, low-fat with sugar, and low fat with sugar substitute.

## Fat List

Butter, margarine, cream, mayonnaise, nuts, salad dressings, vegetable oils, and other fatty foods.

One choice provides:
   5 g fat
   45 calories

### Best for Your Heart and Blood Vessels
   Margarine: soft, tub, or stick
   Mayonnaise: reduced-calorie
   Nuts: almonds, peanuts, walnuts
   Oils: corn, cottonseed, safflower, soy, sunflower, olive,
      peanut
   Olives: green or black
   Salad dressings: French, Italian, mayonnaise-type

### Not as Good for Your Heart and Blood Vessels
   Bacon
   Butter
   Coffee whitener, liquid
   Cool Whip™
   Cream: half-and-half, sour cream
   Cream cheese: whipped or "lite"

## Meat List

Meat, fish, poultry, eggs, cheese, and meat substitutes.

### Low-Fat Protein
One low-fat choice provides:
   3 g fat
   7 g protein
   55 calories

Low-fat choices:

    Cheese: cottage, pot, 1% fat, Lite-Line™, Nuform™,
        Weight Watchers™

    Canned: water-packed salmon or tuna; water-packed clams,
        oysters, scallops, shrimp; sardines, drained

    Fresh or frozen: fish and seafood

    Luncheon meat: 95% fat-free

    Poultry: chicken, turkey, or Cornish hen without skin

### Medium-Fat Protein

One medium-fat choice provides:

    5 g fat

    7 g protein

    75 calories

Medium-fat choices:

    Cheese: skim or part-skim milk cheese; Parmesan,
        Romano

    Beef: chipped, chuck, flank steak, hamburger with
        15% fat, rib eye, rump sirloin, tender-loin top, and bot-
        tom round

    Lamb

    Pork, except for deviled ham, ground pork, and spareribs

    Veal

    Eggs

    Egg Substitutes

### High-Fat Protein

One high-fat choice provides:

    8 g fat

    7 g protein

    100 calories

High-fat choices:

These protein foods are high in fat. Do not use them often.

Regular cheese: blue, Brie, cheddar, Colby feta, Monterey Jack, Muenster, provolone, Swiss, pasteurized process

Fried fish

Beef: brisket, club and rib steaks, corned beef, regular hamburger with 20% fat, rib roast, short ribs

Frankfurters

Luncheon meats: bologna, bratwurst, braunschweiger, knockwurst, liverwurst, pastrami

Organ meats: liver, heart, kidney

Polish sausage, salami

Pork: deviled ham, ground pork, spareribs, sausage (patty or link)

## Starch/Bread List

Bread, crackers, cereal, pasta, starchy vegetables, and other starchy food items.

One choice provides:

trace of fat

15 g carbohydrates

3 g protein

80 calories

### *Breads*

In general, one choice equals 1 ounce of bread.

Bagel

English muffin

Reduced-calorie: (1 slice equals 40 calories)

Rolls: dinner, plain, hamburger

Pitas, 6-inch diameter

White, whole-wheat, or rye

## Cereals

One choice equals ½ cup serving.

Bran: All Bran™, 40 percent
  Bran Flakes™,
  Wheat Chex™
Cooked cereals
Cornflakes™
Nutrigrain™, wheat
Puffed rice or wheat

Rice Krispies™
Shredded Wheat™ biscuit*
  spoon-size
Special K™
Sunflakes™
Wheat Cheerios™

*Cereals high in fiber*

## Starchy Vegetables

Corn
Lima beans
Peas, green, canned or frozen
Potato, white, mashed or baked

Sweet potato,
  mashed or baked
Winter squash:
  acorn or butternut

## Pasta (Cooked)

Macaroni, noodles, spaghetti

## Dried Beans, Peas, and Lentils

Baked beans, canned, no pork (vegetarian style)
Beans, peas, lentils (dried and cooked)

## Prepared Foods

Biscuit, 2-inch diameter (1 ounce)
Cornbread, 2-by-2-by-1 inches
Croissant, 4-by-4-by-1¾ inches
Muffin, bran or corn, 2-inch diameter (1½ ounces)
Pancake, 4-inch diameter
Waffle, 4-inch diameter

### Others
Bread crumbs
Potato or macaroni salad
Rice, cooked

### Occasional Choices
These foods are high in fat. Do not use more than two times a week.

French fries, 2- to 3½-inch length   Popcorn, popped in oil
Ice cream                            Potato or corn chips
Popcorn, microwave                   Stuffing mix, cooked

### Crackers (Equal to One Bread Choice)
Gingersnaps                          Rye Krisp™, three triple
Graham crackers                         crackers
  2½-inch squares          Saltine™ crackers
Matzoh™                              Stella D'Oro Egg Biscuit™
Melba™ toast rectangles              Uneedas™
Pretzel sticks                       Wasa Lite™ or Golden
Rice cakes                              Crisp Bread™

### Crackers (Equal to One Bread Plus One Fat Choice)
These crackers are high in fat. Count them as one bread choice plus one fat choice.

Cheez-its™                           Stella D'Oro Sesame
Club™ or Townhouse™                     Breadsticks™
  crackers                 Triscuits™
Peanut Butter Sandwich               Vanilla Wafers™
  Crackers™                Wasa Sesame™ or
Pepperidge Farm Goldfish™               Breakfast Crisp Bread™
Ritz™                                Wheat Thins™
Stella D'Oro Breakfast
  Treats™

## Vegetable List

Fresh, frozen, and canned vegetables.

One choice provides:

> 5 g carbohydrates
> 2 g protein
> 28 calories

### Vegetables

| | |
|---|---|
| Asparagus | Mushrooms, fresh |
| Beets | Spinach, cooked |
| Broccoli | Squash, summer or zucchini |
| Carrots | Tomato, ripe |
| Cauliflower | Tomato sauce, canned |
| Green beans | Vegetables, mixed |

### Low-Calorie Vegetables

These vegetables are low in calories. Eat them raw and enjoy as much as you want.

| | |
|---|---|
| Alfalfa sprouts | Lettuce |
| Chicory | Parsley |
| Chinese cabbage | Pickles, unsweetened |
| Cucumber | Pimento |
| Endive | Spinach |
| Escarole | Watercress |

## Fruit List

Fresh fruit, pure fruit juices, and canned, dried, cooked, or frozen fruit without extra sugar.

One choice provides:

> 15 g carbohydrates
> 60 calories

*Fruits*

Apple, 2-inch diameter

Banana, 9-inch length

Blueberries

Cantaloupe, 5-inch diameter, sectioned, cubed

Grapefruit, 4-inch diameter

Grapes

Nectarine, 2½-inch diameter

Orange, 3-inch diameter

Peach, 2½-inch diameter, fresh, canned*

Pear, fresh, canned*

Pineapple, canned*

Prunes, dried, medium

Raisins

Strawberries

Tangerine, 2½-inch diameter

Watermelon, diced

*Do not use the liquid from canned fruit.*

## Foods Using More Than One Food Group

*Canned Soup*

Cream soup made with water

Minestrone, ready-to-serve

Rice or noodle with broth prepared with water

Tomato, made with water

*Other Foods*

Beef stew, homemade

Chili with meat and beans, homemade

Plain cheese pizza

Pudding, sugar-free, made with non-fat (skim) or 1% low-
fat milk

Ravioli, canned

## Free Food Group

These foods are low in calories. You may have as much as you want unless otherwise noted.

| | |
|---|---|
| Bouillon cubes | Mustard, prepared |
| Calorie-free soft drinks | Pickles, unsweetened |
| Catsup (1 tablespoon daily) | Soy sauce |
| Coffee | Spices |
| Herbs | Tea |
| Horseradish | Vinegar |

## Foods Likely to Cause Problems

These foods are high in sugar and may cause high blood sugar. Do not use them unless your dietitian or doctor says you can.

Alcohol*: sweet wines, liqueurs, cordials

Candy

Carbonated beverages containing sugar
    (including "natural" sodas)

Chewing gum (regular)

Dates, figs, and other dried fruits

Desserts containing sugar: cakes; cookies with filling or frost-
    ing; ice cream, including sodas and sundaes; ice milk;
    gelatin desserts, sweetened; pies; puddings; sherbet

Fructose

Fruited yogurt

Honey

Jam and jelly (non-dietetic)

Marmalade

Pastries

Preserves

Sugar

Sugar-coated cereals

Sugar-sweetened fruit drinks (Kool-Aid™, Hi-C™, etc.)

Sweetened condensed milk

Syrups (maple, molasses, etc.)

*Avoid all alcohol unless your doctor or dietitian advises otherwise.*
*Source: Presbyterian Diabetes Center of Albuquerque*

## ❧ Appendix F

# A SAMPLE WEEKLY LOG

This is an excerpt from my weekly log over the Christmas holiday. It is not meant to be used as a sample diet for a week. Rather, it is meant to show that diabetics do not have to eat "perfectly" at every meal. I chose this week because we had holiday meals, ate out, went to a party, and also ate leftovers, as most "normal" people do. This menu might make a Certified Diabetes Educator cringe, but it—along with daily exercise—did manage to keep my blood sugar readings under control, which is what diabetics should try to achieve.

### December 24 Christmas Eve

| *Blood Glucose Readings* | | *Exercise Record* | |
|---|---|---|---|
| 7:25 A.M. | 117 | Walk/Treadmill | 1½ miles |
| 5:30 P.M. | 102 | Exercise Bike | 2 miles |
| | | Stairs | 206 |
| | | Stepper | ¼ mile |

*Today's Menu*
Breakfast:          ½ cup Bran Flakes™ and ½ cup
                    Special K™ cereal
                  ½ cup 2% milk
                  1 medium banana

209

Mid-morning snack: 2 vanilla cookies

Lunch: 1 ground beef patty
¾ hamburger bun
12 low-fat potato chips
½ cup vanilla frozen yogurt
1 sugar-free almond cookie

Supper: 1 3-ounce piece of ham
½ cup scalloped potatoes
1 tablespoon baked beans
sugar-free pistachio pudding salad
1 sugar-free cookie

Late evening snack: ½ cup vanilla and strawberry sugar-free
frozen yogurt

## December 25 Christmas Day

| *Blood Glucose Readings* | | *Exercise Record* | |
|---|---|---|---|
| 9 A.M. | 103 | Walk/Treadmill | 1¼ miles |
| 5:50 P.M. | 103 | Exercise Bike | 2 miles |
| | | Stairs | 201 |
| | | Stepper | ½ mile |

*Today's Menu*

Breakfast: ½ cup Bran Flakes™ and ½ cup
Special K™ cereal
½ cup 2% milk
1 large banana

Lunch: I did not "keep track" of portion sizes on
this day, but I ate at every meal and also
had a snack in the evening.

Supper: sirloin steak
mashed potatoes

carrots

whole-wheat rolls

gelatin salad

tossed salad

dessert

Late evening snack: sugar-free cookie

## December 26

### Blood Glucose Readings

| | | Exercise Record | |
|---|---|---|---|
| 8:40 A.M. | 107 | Walk/Treadmill | 1½ miles |
| 5:10 P.M. | 85 | Exercise Bike | 2 miles |
| | | Stairs | 174 |
| | | Stepper | ½ mile |

### Today's Menu

| | |
|---|---|
| Breakfast: | ½ cup Bran Flakes™ and ½ cup Special K™ cereal |
| | ½ cup 2% milk |
| | 1 medium banana |
| Lunch: | 3-ounce steak |
| | ½ cup mashed potatoes |
| | 4 pieces carrots |
| | ½ cup peppermint frozen yogurt |
| | 1 peanut butter sugar-free cookie |
| Supper: | 3 ounces baked ham |
| | 1 slice rye bread |
| | margarine |
| | 14 lite potato chips |
| | sugar-free raspberry frozen yogurt |

Late evening snack: 1 vanilla sugar-free cookie

# December 27

## *Blood Glucose Readings*

| | |
|---|---|
| 7:30 A.M. | 104 |
| 5:30 P.M. | 113 |

## *Exercise Record*

| | |
|---|---|
| Walk/Treadmill | ¾ mile |
| Exercise Bike | 2½ Miles |
| Stairs | 200 |
| Stepper | ½ mile |

## *Today's Menu*

Breakfast:
: ½ cup Bran Flakes™ and ½ cup Special K™ cereal
½ cup 2% milk
1 medium banana

Lunch (ate out with friends):
: ½ Chicken Kiev
tossed salad with lettuce, tomatoes, cucumbers, onions, celery, green peppers, low-fat ranch dressing
½ roll
1 slice sugar-free "coffee bread"
1 peanut butter sugar-free cookie

Supper:
: 1 slice rye bread
fat-free margarine
3 thin slices hickory smoked sausage
1 slice tomato
14 low-fat potato chips
1 tablespoon low-fat sour cream dip
½ cup sugar-free vanilla yogurt

Late evening snack: ½ cup raspberry frozen dessert

# December 28

## Blood Glucose Readings

| | |
|---|---|
| 8:15 A.M. | 106 |
| 5:30 P.M. | 111 |

## Exercise Record

| | |
|---|---|
| Walk/Treadmill | 1 mile |
| Exercise Bike | 2 miles |
| Stairs | 175 |
| Stepper | ¾ mile |

## Today's Menu

Breakfast: ½ cup Bran Flakes™ and ½ cup
Special K™ cereal
½ cup 2% milk
1 medium banana

Lunch: 1 beef hotdog with catsup and mustard
1 hotdog bun
2 slices tomatoes
½ cup raspberry dessert

Supper: ½ cup Beef Stroganoff
1 slice rye bread
2 slices tomatoes
¼ cup mashed potatoes
½ cup gelatin dessert
1 peanut butter sugar-free cookie

Late evening snack: ½ cup raspberry frozen yogurt

# December 29

## Blood Glucose Readings

| | |
|---|---|
| 9:00 A.M. | 113 |
| 5:30 P.M. | 95 |

## Exercise Record

| | |
|---|---|
| Walk/Treadmill | 2 miles |
| Exercise Bike | 2 miles |
| Stairs | 175 |
| Stepper | 0 |

*Today's Menu*

| Breakfast: | ½ cup Bran Flakes™ and ½ cup Special K™ cereal |
|---|---|
| | ½ cup 2% milk |
| | 1 medium banana |
| Lunch: | 1 cup ravioli |
| | sugar-free gelatin |
| Supper (ate out with friends): | ½ cup potato salad |
| | 4 ounces slice turkey breast |
| | tossed salad with lettuce, sliced tomatoes, celery, cucumbers, low-fat ranch dressing, bacon bits, and 1 tablespoon croutons |
| | gelatin salad with raspberries |
| Late evening snack: | ½ cup vanilla sugar-free frozen yogurt |

## December 30

### Blood Glucose Readings

| 8:50 A.M. | 98 |
|---|---|
| 5:20 P.M. | 92 |

### Exercise Record

| Walk/Treadmill | 1 mile |
|---|---|
| Exercise Bike | 2½ miles |
| Stairs | 175 |
| Stepper | ½ mile |

*Today's Menu*

| Breakfast: | ½ cup Bran Flakes™ and ½ cup Special K™ cereal |
|---|---|
| | ½ cup 2% milk |
| | 1 medium banana |
| Lunch: | ½ cup potato salad |
| | 2 ounces turkey breast |
| | 2 slices tomatoes |
| | ½ cup vanilla sugar-free pudding |

Supper:                4 ounces meatloaf
                       ½ cup mashed potatoes
                       1 teaspoon low-fat margarine
                       ½ cup sugar-free gelatin with strawberries
                       1 almond sugar-free cookie
Late evening snack:    2 tablespoons gelatin and low-fat dessert
                       topping

## December 31

### Blood Glucose Readings

| 9:00 A.M. | 95 |
| 5:10 P.M. | 102 |

### Exercise Record

| Walk/Treadmill | 1 mile |
| Exercise Bike | 2½ miles |
| Stairs | 177 |
| Stepper | ½ mile |

### Today's Menu

Breakfast:             ½ cup Bran Flakes™ and ½ cup
                       Special K™ cereal
                       ½ cup 2% milk
                       1 medium banana
Lunch:                 1 cup chili con carne
                       6 club crackers
                       1 sugar-free peanut butter cookie
Supper (New Year's     6 ounces prime rib
Eve, ate out with      1 medium baked potato
friends):              low-fat sour cream
                       tossed salad with lettuce, tomato,
                           cucumber, celery, green pepper, carrots,
                           low-calorie ranch dressing
                       1 whole-wheat roll
                       margarine

Late evening snack: ½ cup party mix
　　　　　　　　　1 piece sugar-free coffee bread
　　　　　　　　　½ cup frozen dessert

## January 1 Happy Healthy New Year

*Blood Glucose Readings*

7:50 A.M.　　　92

# GLOSSARY

**Bake:**   Cook in oven.

**Beat:**   Stir briskly, around and around vertically.

**Blend:**   Mix two or more ingredients together.

**Chop:**   Cut into small pieces with a chopper or knife.

**Cream:**   Beat into a creamy, light, and fluffy consistency, such as combining shortening and eggs.

**Dash:**   Less than ⅛ teaspoon of any ingredient.

**Dice:**   Cut into very small pieces.

**Dust:**   Sprinkle pan lightly with flour.

**Dutch Oven:**   Large heavy cooking kettle with tight fitting cover.

**Fold:**   Combine ingredients together gently, bringing spoon through a mixture, across bottom, and up sides of bowl. Broader and slower than beating.

**Free Food:**   Any food that has fewer than 20 calories.

**Frozen Yogurt:**   Combine plain, regular, or non-fat yogurt with fruit or other flavorings and sweeteners to make a tangy frozen dessert.

**Ice Cream:**   Flavored frozen cream with air whipped into it. Commercial ice cream contains 20 percent milk solids by weight, using cream, half-and-half, or a combination of these and often contain eggs and has a high cholesterol and fat content.

**Ice Milk:**   Uses milk instead of cream, with 1 percent milk solids. Ice milk has less fat and calorie content than ice cream. By making ice milk, you can control the calories and fat by using 2 percent or whole milk.

**Knead:**   Use hands to work dough.

**Marinate:**   Let ingredients stand in a liquid for 2 or more hours to enhance flavors.

**Mash:**   Stir or use masher to make a soft mass.

**Mince:**   Chop very fine. (Diced is finer than chopped; minced is finer than diced.)

**Puree:**   Place cooked food into a blender or pressed through a sieve into a smooth consistency.

**Sherbet:**   Combination of milk, fruit or fruit juice, and sweeteners. Unflavored gelatin or whipped egg whites may be used to give a lighter texture.

**Shred:**   Tear or cut into small pieces.

**Simmer:**   Cook in liquid over low heat without boiling.

**Sorbets:**   Use pureed fruit or fruit juice frozen and aerated with a simple sugar and water syrup. Make non-sweet sorbets by using water-based recipes.

**Tester:**   Cake tester, toothpick, or knife inserted into the middle of breads or cakes to test for doneness.

**Toss:**   Mix lightly.

**Whip:**   Beat rapidly to increase volume as in whipping egg whites.

**Whisk:**   An implement used to mix with a back and forth, round and round motion (also called a wire whip).

# INDEX